With *Thai Massage,* Ananda Apfelbaum has made an important contribution by capturing this sacred healing art with clarity and precision. It presents a comprehensive overview followed by a clearly illustrated, complete, full-body Thai massage sequence. I highly recommend this book to anyone interested in experiencing the tremendous benefits and joy of this ancient practice.

JONAS WESTRING, *physical therapist and director of Thai Yoga Healing Arts*

It's gratifying to come across such an approachable and methodical guidebook for learning the sacred art of Thai massage. Throughout her book, Ananda never loses sight of the real focus of her work—compassion for others. Every therapist could glean something from this story.

STEPHAN RECHTSCHAFFEN, *cofounder and CEO of The Omega Institute for Holistic Studies*

In this meticulously researched book, Ananda Apfelbaum places traditional Thai massage in its cultural context. She skillfully weaves together the influences of India and China to illuminate the unique quality of this ancient and powerful form of bodywork. She offers precise instruction on how to move through sequences developed by master healer Pichest Boonthumme, never forgetting that the most important ingredient in a successful treatment is compassion. This book is an important contribution to preserving an oral tradition that has had little written documentation.

LORI BRUNGARD, *codirector of Ashtanga Yoga Shala, NYC*

Fortunately for contemporary culture, the ancients evolved methods for attuning to the healing powers of the life force, known in yoga as "prana." Thai massage embodies this tradition in a ritualized way that enhances well-being and produces deeply relaxed states of being. Ananda transmits both the technique and the spirit of Thai massage through her sensitive abilities to teach and inspire. The book is a wonderful doorway through time to reconnect with primal wisdom.

DON STAPLETON, PhD, *codirector of Nosara Yoga Institute and Interdisciplinary Yoga Teacher Training*

Ananda has done a masterful job of translating her passion, consummate skill, and the essence of Thai massage into words for this book. . . . A must for massage schools and bodyworkers of all types and levels.

WILL POLEC, NMD (Naturopathic Medical Doctor)

THAI MASSAGE

ANANDA
APFELBAUM

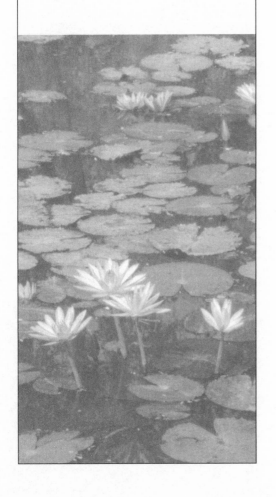

THAI

MASSAGE

Sacred Bodywork

Avery

a member of

Penguin Group (USA) Inc.

New York

a member of
Penguin Group (USA) Inc.
375 Hudson Street
New York, NY 10014
www.penguin.com

Copyright © 2004 by Ananda Apfelbaum
Line illustrations by Tan Waphat, Joan Berry, and Ananda Apfelbaum
Maps by Henry Kaufman
Interior photographs of Thai massage techniques by Anna Isaak-Ross
An additional list of photo credits appears on page 258.
Thai massage techniques demonstrated by Ananda Apfelbaum and Pichest Boonthumme (practitioners) and Ganitha Manepakorn Notman and Helena de-Leeuw (models)

Library of Congress Cataloging-in-Publication Data

Apfelbaum, Ananda.
    Thai massage : sacred bodywork / Ananda Apfelbaum.
        p.   cm.
    Includes bibliographical references.
    ISBN 1-58333-168-9 (alk. paper)
    1. Massage therapy—Thailand.   2. Medicine, Thai.   I. Title.
    RM723.T45A64   2003   2003056263
    615.8'22'09593—dc21

Printed in the United States of America
10   9   8   7   6   5   4   3   2   1

This book is printed on acid-free paper. ♾

Book design by Lee Fukui

This book is dedicated to my Thai massage teacher,
Ahjarn Pichest Boonthumme,
with tremendous gratitude for all that he has taught me,
for his friendship and for his true spirit as a healer;
and to my spiritual teacher,
His Holiness The Dalai Lama,
with tremendous reverence for inspiring me along
the path of wisdom and compassion.

CONTENTS

PART II

THE PRACTICE

*If we think carefully, from a wider perspective we owe
our entire present and future collection of good qualities
to the kindness of sentient beings. When you are strongly
motivated to work for others, you can lead a meaningful life.
When you have a strong inclination to benefit others,
you will find that you are always happy.*

—His Holiness The Dalai Lama

THAI MASSAGE

THE
BACKGROUND

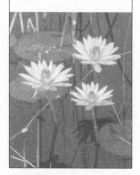

Water Lilies at Sukhothai

*In general, Shakyamuni Buddha taught doctrines in accordance
with the predispositions and interests of trainees; among these
doctrines, the science of medicine is particularly supreme. The
reason for this is that, for instance, ordinarily the six perfections
of giving, ethics, patience, effort, concentration, and wisdom
cannot immediately be practiced simultaneously and instead are
practiced one by one, but, with medicine, once its essentials have
been realized and put into practice, the six perfections are
accomplished simultaneously.*

—Dr. Yeshi Dhonden

MASSAGE: COMPASSION IN ACTION

What greater gift can one give than the gift of love? Massage is a perfect vehicle through which to express this love. It transcends all borders, touching not only the physical body but also the heart and mind. It expresses care and kindness in a way that is so direct that it can be absorbed immediately.

Touch was our first language of communication. Even in the womb we were affected by touch, and then as a baby and young child this continued to be our main means of communication. Studies show that premature babies who are touched grow and develop almost two times as fast as premature babies without touch.

In his book, *Where Healing Waters Meet: Touching Mind and Emotion Through the Body* (Station Hill Press, 1989), chiropractor and therapist Clyde W. Ford wrote, "Touch . . . creates a powerful therapeutic alliance, so vital to the healing process. Reaching out to touch someone is a lasting symbol of what it means to be human, and a universal sign of healing . . . when we touch, the human factor is unavoidable—in fact, it becomes the central aspect of healing."[1]

The use of touch for healing goes back thousands of years. Healing touch seems to have existed under different names among all ancient cultures. It was used long before people knew just why it had such beneficial effects and seems to arise spontaneously when we see someone in pain. From touch, massage evolved, and later came healing sciences such as acupuncture and surgery. Knowledge was passed down from generation to generation. The oldest written reference to therapeutic massage found so far is in China's *The Yellow Emperor's Classic of Internal Medicine* and in *Cong-Fou of the Tao-Tse,* which dates back 3,000 years. Other references dating back 2,500 years can be found in Indian Ayurvedic literature.

Massage therapy heals on physical, psychological, and spiritual levels. In fact, it is so powerful that it can boost the body's immune system and is capable of increasing levels of serotonin—the same neurotransmitter that responds to the antidepressant Prozac.

In massage, the ability to touch others truly has both a figurative and a literal meaning. It is a tremendous vehicle through which to express one's compassion and to expand one's heart out to others. I remember many years ago when I was feeling frustrated by my work as a massage therapist, I went to a Tibetan lama to discuss this. He looked at me and said simply, "How fortunate you are to be doing compassionate work. At least you needn't have any conflict about the kind of work you do." As my work proceeds, I hold this in my heart and let my hands speak this message. May this book help you to learn a sacred form of massage that was deeply influenced by the Buddha, most compassionate of beings.

CHAPTER

2

MASSAGE: EAST AND WEST

The greater a person's heart realization of true Dharma, the greater a doctor he can be, for he will have the two-fold Buddha nature aspects of wisdom and compassion, rendering him more capable of understanding the depths of the medical science and serving the physical, emotional and spiritual needs of his patients.

—TERRY CLIFFORD

Eastern and Western massage have very different approaches to the body based on the health philosophies of their cultures. Western massage focuses mainly on the external physical body. It does not perceive an internal energy flow. Its goal is to make the physical body as comfortable as possible. Eastern massage, on the other hand, such as Thai massage, goes beyond this by also considering the energy flow within the body. Its goal is to restore the whole person, both external and internal, to a state of balance. Let's look at these contrasting goals by examining Eastern and Western views on health, which form the backbone of their healing approaches. In the West, health has been defined as good unless there are physical signs that something isn't functioning well. The body and mind are viewed as separate entities, and even parts within the body are held separately. The body is purely a physical organism without an energetic component. It is approached from a scientific, "objective" point of view, with the focus on tangible physical structures such as organs, bones, and muscles. Any malfunction is viewed mechanically, as a separate entity. The instant cure is looked for and marveled at. People are assumed to be more or less the same, so individualized treatment approaches aren't necessary. In cases of chronic illness, diagnosis of the body's internal functions is usually defined in terms of deficiency or excess. The condition is then treated, usually through the administration of an externally produced synthetic chemical. The original condition that caused the symptoms in the first place isn't treated. The body becomes lazy, leading to further illness. Health in the West is dealt with by initiating treatment after the onset of disease rather than through long-term prevention. The doctor is in power and the patient is a passive recipient.

In the East, on the other hand, there is a much more comprehensive understanding of health and the body. Health is considered good if there is a balance within the physical, emotional, and spiritual bodies. These three spheres are considered inseparable, interconnected, and energy-based. The whole person is treated with the aim of strengthening their own healing energy. "Health" is believed to be an ongoing process of right lifestyle. It is understood that no one is born with perfect health and so each person must be diligent in maintaining and/or improving his or her health. Diagnosis is made early on as a preventive measure with suggestions for daily living. The uniqueness of each person is cherished and supported. If ill health does occur, the underlying imbalance is looked for in the whole person and harmony reestablished throughout. In an ongoing doctor-patient relationship, the doctor is held responsible for not catching an illness early on.

Thai medical philosophy, like other Eastern medical philosophies, stresses the indivisible interdependence of mind, body, and vitality. It advocates treating the whole person and not just a particular symptom. It is based on the holistic point of view that any problem is not simply an illness of a particular part, but rather a disorder of the whole being. All parts of the body are believed to have an organic relationship that exists within an even greater whole—nature. Due to this holistic approach, Thai massage treatments are usually two to three hours long so that a person's whole body can be addressed and not just a "problem" area. Furthermore, the Thai people believe that for optimal results, Thai massage should be used along with good diet, spiritual practices, and, if necessary, medicine.

Pichest Boonthumme (pronounced Pih-ched Bun-thum-me), whose style this book is based on, always points out the connections between one problem area and another in the body, thus demonstrating that nothing exists in isolation. He also indicates energy lines that are out of balance as he rebalances them and sometimes, based on his psychic ability, speaks of the person's spiritual or emotional problems and what can be done to heal them. Wataru Ohashi, renowned shiatsu teacher, reinforces these ideas in his book *Do-It-Yourself Shiatsu* (Penguin USA, 2001) when he says, "In the Orient we believe you are built in one piece, that it is impossible to isolate a part without considering what effect it will have on the whole. We do not concentrate on the illness, but on the entire body. We do not label disease, because all diseases come from the same source—an imbalance of energy flow throughout the body."[1]

THAI MASSAGE:
A UNIQUE STYLE

*To help others is the most effective way possible we have to be
fully enlightened buddhas.*

—HIS HOLINESS THE DALAI LAMA

Thai massage is a unique style of massage based upon the principles of compassion. It is one of the four branches of traditional Thai medicine, which are manipulation, medicine (orals, salves, compresses, and vapors), diet, and spiritual ceremonies or magical practices. As mentioned earlier, Thai massage, which falls under the branch of manipulation, should be practiced in conjunction with the three other branches of traditional Thai medicine for the most comprehensive results.

Thai massage is an amazing synthesis of many techniques—leaning pressure, reflexology, energy line work, blood stopping, stretching, and yoga. To achieve all of these effects, Thai massage therapists use more parts of their bodies to give a massage than therapists in any other modality. They use their palms, thumbs, feet, elbows, forearms, and knees. The receiver is moved through a wide variety of postures within five positions—supine, side lying, prone, inverted, and seated. The work is done on a mat on the floor. If anyone claims to do Thai massage on a table, he or she is not doing it properly, because it cannot be done effectively that way. Thai massage has to be done on a mat on the floor where there is plenty of room to move around and where the therapist can use his or her "center" over, behind, or to the side of the recipient. (More information about the use of one's center will be found in Chapter 7.)

In any case, Thai massage is an ancient healing technique and not a cover-up for a sexual experience in a "massage parlor." It is a genuine form of bodywork with a very ancient and honorable tradition.

In fact, many people believe that Thai massage originated in India and that it was brought over to Thailand 2,500 years ago. If this was the case, it still must have mixed with indigenous as well as Chinese forms of massage after it arrived. Others believe that it was an indigenous form of massage that was influenced by Indian and Chinese massage, and still others believe that it developed solely out of Chinese massage. Whatever the case, there was not much contact between different parts of Thailand long ago due to the fact that there were few roads and many difficult-to-traverse mountains, forests, and jungles. Thai massage therefore developed differently from region to region. Even within each region, there were different styles due to different traditions being kept within families or temples. Furthermore, due to the absence of literacy, the tradition was predominantly passed down orally. Therefore, there was no widespread dissemination of literature, which could have had a unifying effect. Nowadays, however, due to increased literacy and travel between all parts of Thailand, the differences between the various styles are decreasing.

There are four main styles of Thai massage: the northern, the central, the southern, and the northeastern. The northern and central styles are more widely known than the others outside of Thailand. The northern style, which Pichest Boonthumme practices, is very dynamic. It uses more stretching than the other styles. In the north, the main school and treatment center is the Old Medicine Hospital in Chiangmai. It is a very popular place, and in the winter (the optimal time to be in the north), classes are filled to capacity with many foreign students. In central Thailand, the main school and treatment center is at Wat Pho temple in Bangkok. Classes there are one on one or group classes. Following is an introduction to the techniques used in Thai massage.

LEANING PRESSURE

Leaning pressure is one of the most important techniques behind effective Thai massage. It is also used in shiatsu. What exactly is leaning pressure? It is a relaxed yet firm and focused leaning that enables the practitioner's whole body weight to go through to the receiver. Unlike muscular exertion, leaning pressure enables the recipient's body to open up to receive the healing impact of the pressure and allows his or her own healing energy to move toward balance. This strongly contrasts with forceful pressure, which causes the receiver's body to tighten up in an attempt to shield itself. Although one does have to be strong to do this kind of work, muscular force should not generally be used. Also, by using leaning pressure, energy flow between the practitioner and the recipient is facilitated.

In order for this technique to work, the surface under the receiver must be firm enough to support the practitioner's pressure. If the surface is too soft, there will not be enough resistance to the pressure and the technique will not work. (A detailed explanation of how to apply leaning pressure will be found in Chapter 7.)

REFLEXOLOGY

The feet are worked on a lot in Thai massage. The large number of nerve endings and reflex points on the feet make them very responsive to touch. That, combined with their noninvasive location, makes them an ideal location to work on. Furthermore, foot work has a profound grounding and relaxing effect that is essential in treating stress—the leading component behind illness. The main techniques used in Thai foot massage are joint mobilization and a modified version of reflexology.

Reflexology is believed to have been practiced by the Chinese, the Indians, the Incas, the Native Americans, the Egyptians, and other groups for thousands of years. The oldest evidence of it found so far is on an Egyptian tomb drawing dating back to between 2500 and 2300 B.C.E. that shows two people receiving reflexology.

Reflexology uses pressure to work on reflex points, which are found on the feet, hands, ears, and irises of the eyes. A reflex point is a point that is connected with a distant body part. When reflex points (excluding those in the eyes, of course) are pressed, energy mysteriously flows to their corresponding body parts. No one knows exactly how this happens, although energy pathways are often credited. Some reflexologists say that pressure activates an electrochemical nerve impulse that is transmitted to the central nervous system, and ganglia (groups of nerve cells that form nerve centers) in turn transmit a message, causing a response. The body's inherent healing potential is stimulated and physiological change takes place.

In reflexology, each foot represents half of the body, with the right foot representing the right side of the body and the left foot representing the left side. The reflex areas on the feet are as follows:

- The toes correspond with the head.

- The balls of the feet correspond with the chest.

- The insteps correspond with the internal organs.

- The heels correspond with the pelvis.

- The medial (inner) sides of the feet correspond with the spine.

- The lateral (outer) sides of the feet correspond with the limbs, hips, and shoulders.

For a detailed depiction of these correspondences, see Figures 3.1 and 3.2. These correspondences also hold true for the hands.

In the traditional medical systems of India and China—both of which, as mentioned before, seem to have been involved with the development of Thai massage—the feet, the hands, and their connected energy pathways are very important. In fact, Ayurveda, which is India's traditional medical form, speaks of *nadis* (channels) that run to the feet and hands, which have energy openings to the external world. In Ayurveda, each of the five fingers is related to one of the traditional five elements. Similarly, in traditional Chinese medicine (TCM), the twelve main meridians (energy pathways), all of which are connected with internal organs, go to the tips of the toes and fingers. In fact, as one book on Thai manual medicine puts it, "The connection with the fingers and toes provided in *sen kaalathaarii* in the

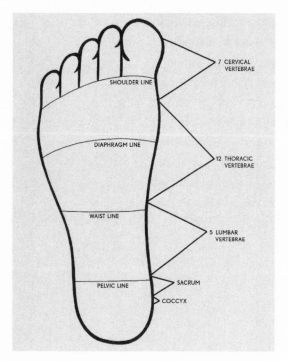

Figure 3.1: The Foot's Correspondences with the Body

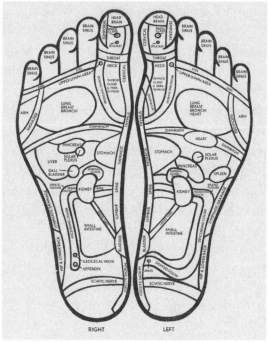

Figure 3.2: Reflexology Areas of the Feet

Thai system is broadly similar to the peripheral linkage with the fingers and toes in the Chinese jing-luo [channels and collaterals] system."[1]

ENERGY LINES

Thai massage uses energy line work on the body. This is based on the Eastern understanding that energy forms the basis of all life and that this energy travels along invisible pathways within the body. In ancient India, holy men known as *rishis* meditated at the foothills of the Himalayas. Over time, they developed the power to see this energy and trace its pathways. Ancient healers in Thailand either discovered these pathways on their own or adopted them from India's and/or China's traditional medical systems.

What is this energy? Different cultures have given different names to this energy. In India, it is called *prana;* in China, *chi* (or *qi*); in Japan, *ki;* and in Thailand, *lom,* which means "wind." This energy can be defined as vital force. It is absorbed from the air we breathe and the food we eat, and is believed to move within us along invisible pathways. In Thailand, these pathways are called *sen;* in India, *nadis;* in China and Japan, *meridians, channels,* and/or *vessels;* and in Tibet, *channels.* In India, which is where many Eastern healing arts—including those of Thailand and Tibet—originated, there are said to be 72,000 nadis. It is not surprising, therefore, to find that Thailand and Tibet also recognize exactly the same number of energy lines. According to *Tibetan Buddhist Medicine and Psychiatry* (Samuel Weiser, 1984), it is said that in Tibet the "[the energy lines] are sometimes numbered 72,000, but are also said to be uncountable."[2] Whatever the number of lines, where they run and what they do varies ". . . depending on the medical system . . . involved. They are not solid realities which one can point out like in the physical body, in spite of the fact that people often try to make exact identifications with particular parts of the body. Such identifications do not hold up. There are, however, more general correspondences which do have meaning and significance."[3] These pathways, according to shiatsu practitioner and teacher Ryokyu Endo, ". . . can be felt only through personal experience and therefore belong to a world indefinable by words. Clinically, the position and depth of meridians varies infinitely according to each patient. . . . Because of their qualitative nature, meridians can only be perceived by an equally qualitative mind. Healers are able to recognize meridians when they are in sympathy with the patient's vital energies and there is a fusion between the feelings of the two. . . . In fact, meridians cannot be understood outside the concept and practice of curing the patient through the touch of the skin . . ."[4]

The energy lines used in Thai massage are worked equally up and down, unlike in shiatsu, where they are worked on in a particular direction depending on the effect desired. The philosophy behind the Thai approach is that going up and down the lines clears all obstructions, facilitating unhindered energy flow within the body. Disease is believed to be the result of a blockage in energy flow. (A detailed discussion of the sen will be found in Chapter 5.)

Blood Stopping

Blood stopping is a technique often used in Thai massage that is not found in any other form of massage. In this technique, the practitioner applies pressure to a major artery. This blocks the flow of blood through that artery, causing an increase in arterial pressure above the blockage. The baroreceptors (pressure receptors located in various parts of the heart and circulatory system) sense the increased pressure. They send a message to the heart that induces it to decrease its rate of contraction in order to bring the pressure back to where it used to be. When the blockage is released, a rush of fresh blood engorges the tissues. This rush of blood carries oxygen and nutrients to the cells and helps to remove waste products and toxins.

Why is this technique so popular in Thailand? To get a clue, one must first notice the language that the Thai people use to describe stopping the blood and releasing it. They call it *opening the wind,* with "wind" representing energy. Interestingly, we find that the English word *artery* also was connected with wind. *Artery* comes from the Greek word *arteria,* which literally means "windpipe." As *Taber's Cyclopedic Medical Dictionary* (F. A. Davis Company, 1985) explains, "The ancients believed that air circulated through them from which supposition the name, artery, was derived."[5] So in Thailand, *opening the wind* means enabling energy to flow more freely in the body. Through this flow, greater health can be established. The Thais also believe that stopping and subsequently releasing the blood causes old blood to be exchanged for new blood.

Stopping the blood is traditionally done several times during the massage. It is applied at the femoral and brachial arteries (the main arteries in the thigh and upper arm, respectively). The effect is much more pronounced at the femoral artery than at the brachial artery. Usually the blood is stopped for sixty pulses and then there is a momentary lightening of the pressure. The pressure is then applied again for sixty pulses. The length and number of times the blood is stopped depends on the condition of the individual being treated. For example, the stiffer a person's back is, the longer it is recommended to stop the blood at their femoral artery. This is because blood stopping deeply relaxes the body in preparation for any adjustment given later on. For a stiff back, it is even recommended to stop the blood for as long as one hundred pulses done five times. Stopping the blood at the femoral artery is also recommended for knee pain. As any injury is usually accompanied by impaired or restricted blood flow, stopping and then releasing the blood counteracts this by increasing blood flow to the area, bringing in nutrients and oxygen and helping in the removal of toxins.

Stopping the blood also enables the individual being treated to move into an altered state. I have noticed that even very talkative people become quiet during this time, and many doze off. This makes sense, as the heart doesn't work as hard during the blood stop since the baroreceptors have told it to slow down; this has a relaxing effect. People seem to become more receptive to the massage from this point on.

The way in which people experience blood stopping and release varies widely. During it, some people feel tingling or numbness. This signals that the blood flow has been cut off for too long and that release is overdue. After the release, some people feel a wave of warmth, while others feel cold, and some feel nothing at all.

Pichest Boonthumme, whose massage style this book is based on, often uses the blood stop as a special time to tune into the receiver's life. He sits quietly on the receiver's extended leg, with the receiver in a side-lying position, and closes his eyes. After he finishes, he often surprises the receiver by sharing very private and personal things he picked up about the receiver's life. At other times, the mischievous side of him surfaces and he uses the blood stop as a time to chat or read his mail.

Stopping the blood is contraindicated (not advised) for people with any type of heart and/or blood-vessel disorders, including high blood pressure and varicose veins, as well as for people with diabetic neuropathy.

STRETCHING

Stretching simply means increasing the range of motion. When a muscle is "stretched," it is actually lengthened. In Thai massage, the muscles, tissues, joints, and limbs of the body are taken through their full range of movement. When the stretching is increased progressively and with the help of a therapist, it is called *assisted progressive stretching*. This technique is used extensively in Thai massage. The recipient is put into a posture that stretches some part of the body. The posture is then relaxed only to be repeated again, with the stretch intensified. In between stretches, there is a return to a more relaxed position. The progressive stretching helps to establish greater flexibility. The muscles and connective tissue surrounding the muscle fibers are restructured to attain a greater resting length. The joints' range of motion is increased and muscle soreness is reduced, which is especially helpful after exercise.

In Thai massage, the assisted progressive stretching is usually done as a series of three. After the series of three is done, another posture is used that goes through the same process of assisted progressive stretching—and so on. For example, the person being treated is asked to lie on his or her back with legs up and knees bent. The practitioner stabilizes the position by putting his or her own knees on the person's thighs and then holds the person's heels. The heels are pushed forward until some stretch is felt. The heels are then released enough so that the stretch sensation ceases. The stretch is then repeated, although this time it is a little stronger. This is followed by relaxation of the stretch, and so forth.

One critical aspect of assisted progressive stretching is the rate at which it is done. It must be done slowly in order to allow the muscle enough time to lengthen rather than to shorten, which happens in response to the type of rapid stretching known as *ballistic stretching*. Assisted progressive stretching also allows the practitioner to feel exactly where the edge is—where the discomfort begins—and to ease into that. This is important for preventing injury and it means being really tuned in to the person you are treating. Furthermore, stretches should only be done after the area involved has been warmed up through palming and thumbing.

Thai massage uses a great variety of movements to stretch all the major muscle groups, increasing the body's flexibility and mobility and bringing a wonderful sense of aliveness. The stretching also facilitates the movement of energy throughout the body's energetic pathways.

YOGA

In Thailand, Thai massage is often called the "lazy person's yoga," because the receiver can simply relax while someone else puts them through various postures! What is yoga and how does it work? In *The Sivananda Companion to Yoga* (Simon & Schuster, 1983), Lucy Lidell describes it this way: "Yoga is a complete science of life that originated in India many thousands of years ago. It is the oldest system of personal development in the world, encompassing body, mind and spirit."[6] There are four branches of yoga—Karma, Bhakti, Jnana, and Raja. All of them aspire toward spiritual development and, ultimately, self-realization.

In the West, Raja yoga is the most well-known branch. It involves the transformation of physical and mental control into spiritual energy. Within Raja yoga, there is a subdivision known as Hatha yoga. Hatha yoga uses *asanas*, also known as postures, and *pranayama*, which is breath regulation, to work on the entire body. The spine and joints are mobilized and the muscles, glands, and internal organs are toned. Not only is the physical body rejuvenated, but also the energetic body. The nadis (energy pathways) are activated so that prana (life force) can flow more freely through the body.

In Thai massage, asanas are used, but they are not held for extended periods of time as they are in Hatha yoga. The effect is therefore not as strong. The focus in Thai massage is more on the flow of the whole treatment rather than on the holding of a particular posture. It is significant to point out here that although the asanas are used differently in Thai massage, the very fact that they are part of the routine again gives credibility to the idea that Thai massage had its roots in ancient India. Furthermore, the aim of asana practice, which is to be able to sit comfortably for long periods of time in order to meditate, seems to be echoed in Thai massage, where the treatment sequence actually ends with the recipient in a sitting position. Although it is not required that one should then meditate, this may either be a lost part of the philosophy or it may be assumed that this will automatically happen at the close of a successful treatment. I certainly have seen people at the end of a session look very transformed and serene, and as if they were ready to begin meditating.

COMPRESSES

In Thailand, herbal compresses are sometimes used in addition to massage. The herbs are placed in small bags, which are then warmed by steam. The heated bag is pressed on the body. After it cools down, it is replaced by another warm bag. It is a most relaxing and nurturing sensation. The technique of patting the herb bags on the body is called *prakhob.* This is an example of combining medicine with manipulation—two of the branches of Thai massage.

The most commonly used herbs are cassumunar, camphor, borneol camphor, kiffer lime, lemongrass, turmeric, sweet flag rhizome, and *Acacia concinna.* They stimulate blood circulation in the body and are especially helpful for relieving muscle inflammation, pain, bruising, fatigue, cramping, and muscular atrophy in people who have difficulty moving or exercising.

THE HISTORICAL ROOTS OF THAI MASSAGE

*The task of man is to help others; that's my firm teaching, that's
my message. That is my own belief. For me, the fundamental
question is better relations, better relations among human
beings—and whatever I can contribute to that.*

—His Holiness The Dalai Lama

I t is important to take a look at the historical roots of Thai massage, as
they have affected the development of this unique style. Unfortunately,
since most of the information about Thai massage has been passed down
orally, it is impossible to accurately know its earlier history. Much can be
surmised, however, by examining Thailand's earlier history, as well as India's and China's, as the two latter countries played an important role in the
development of Thai massage.

THAILAND'S BEGINNING

There are many theories on Thailand's early history—who the Thai people
were and where they lived. There is evidence that parts of Thailand were already inhabited 10,000 years ago.

Many scholars say that, based on linguistic theory, the Thais came from
southern China and northern Vietnam. Others, following the development

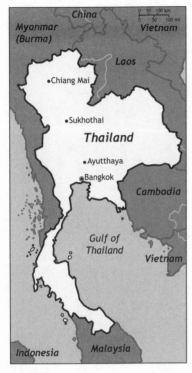

Figure 4.1:
Modern Thailand

of symbols and myths in Thai culture and art, believe that they came from an ocean-based civilization in the western Pacific. A third group postulates that Thai people were indigenous to Thailand. And a fourth group holds that it was peopled through successive migrations from central Asia. Whatever the case, today in Thailand there is an ethnically mixed population, with Thais being the majority (75 percent) followed by people of Chinese stock (14 percent) and then Indian, Malay, Lao, Burmese, Mon, and Khmer populations (11 percent).

According to *Asia, East by South: A Cultural Geography* (John Wiley & Sons, 1954), "The political region today recognized as Thailand has gone through a complex regional history. Though the Menam Valley [Thailand's fertile central region] is the heart of modern Thailand, and though the Thais are the dominant culture group, this is a rather recent development. Earlier cultures and political states were arranged on quite different regional lines."[1] I will not go into all the border changes that occurred under different kingdoms. Suffice it to say that present-day Thailand occupies a central position on the Southeast Asian peninsula. It is the only Southeast Asian country that was never taken over by a European power. On the west and northwest, it is bordered by Myanmar (formerly Burma), on the east and northeast by Laos, on the southeast by Cambodia, and on the south by Malaysia and the Gulf of Thailand. (See Figure 4.1.)

SEA ROUTE AND SILK ROAD

Looking at Thailand's history, it is obvious that the great civilizations of India and China had an impact on Thai culture. Since Thailand is located near these two countries, this is not surprising. India and China's influence on Thailand, however, had more to do with their trading and missionary activity than with proximity. As early as the first century C.E., great maritime trading routes existed between southeast India, Sri Lanka, southeast Asia (including Thailand), and southern China.

There was also the famous overland Silk Road between China and Eu-

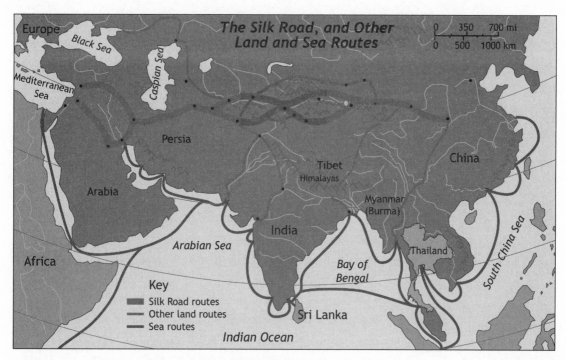

Figure 4.2: The Silk Road, and Other Land and Sea Routes

rope, which flourished from the 100s B.C.E. to the 1500s C.E. The Silk Road—which actually was a "constantly shifting network of pathways for many types of exchanges"[2]—spanned about 7,000 miles, running from eastern China through central Asia and the Middle East to the Mediterranean Sea. Land routes to various countries branched off from the Silk Road. (See Figure 4.2.) The two most significant routes in terms of the development of Thai massage were the routes between India and the Silk Road and between Myanmar (Burma), Thailand's neighbor to the west, and the Silk Road. The Silk Road, besides being a route for trade and migration, was the major vehicle that spread Buddhism throughout Central Asia. Contained within Buddhism was India's precious medical system of Ayurveda. Many of the traders, travelers, and missionaries along the Silk Road also went to Thailand. This had a tremendous impact on Thailand's healthcare system.

The Intertwining of Ayurveda and Buddhism

Ayurveda, which literally means "the science of life," began in India more than 3,000 years ago, when Hinduism and a strong yogic culture were flourishing there. Ayurveda reached its zenith, however, between 500 B.C.E. and 800 C.E., when Buddhism was flourishing in India. Many Hindu Indian men were so moved by the teachings of the Buddha that they became Buddhist monks and practiced Ayurveda as a way of expressing their compassionate care for others.

In the second century B.C.E., 200 years after the Buddha had died, the great Indian emperor Ashoka became a convert to Buddhism. He was so inspired by the Buddha's teachings that he wanted them to reach people everywhere. He therefore sent Buddhist monks abroad. Some traveled to Southeast Asia, settling in Sri Lanka, Thailand, Myanmar, Laos, and Cambodia. During this time, the teachings were brought to a land called *Suvannabhumi*, which means "land of gold." Suvannabhumi seems to have stretched from what is now southern Myanmar across central Thailand to eastern Cambodia. Other monks traveled north and east of India, through Nepal and the Himalayas to Tibet, China, Korea, Mongolia, Vietnam, and Japan. Over time, the form of Buddhism practiced in Southeast Asia became known as Theravada Buddhism and the form practiced in the north and east of India became known as Mahayana Buddhism. Many of these missionary monks practiced Ayurveda. They acted as a kind of "Peace Corps" giving service not only through religious instruction, but also through medical aid, which included the use of medicinal herbs. Wherever the monks went, they built not only temples, but also hospitals and dispensaries. Over time, Ayurveda became integrated with the local medical practices of whichever country the missionaries settled in.

By the twelfth century C.E., Buddhism was in decline in India. Ayurveda, however, remained strong there until the beginning of the twentieth century C.E., when Western medicine began to gradually replace Ayurveda. It was only after India's independence that Ayurveda experienced a resurgence with the backing of the national government. In 1980, the Indian National Congress decided that Ayurveda should be given status equal to that of Western medicine. Since then, they have backed research projects and institutions connected with Ayurveda and it is once again being widely practiced throughout India as well as in Sri Lanka. Ayurveda has also recently been gaining popularity internationally.

THE BUDDHA

Despite the decline of Buddhism in India, it took a strong hold wherever the missionaries went and is still widely practiced throughout most of Asia. Who was the Enlightened One and what was his message?

The Buddha was born as Siddhartha Gautama, son of King Suddhodana, in 564 B.C.E. in Lumbini, India, which is now in Nepal. When Siddhartha was born, there were many signs that he was destined to become a great universal king or an enlightened renunciate (a person who has renounced the secular world). His father—knowing this, and hoping he would become the former—surrounded him with all the luxuries of a princely life. He also tried to prevent his son from experiencing or seeing any kind of suffering. When Siddhartha was sixteen, his father married him off to a young woman named Yashodhara, hoping that this would further distract him from his possible destiny as a renunciate.

Fate arranged otherwise. Just after Yashodhara gave birth to their first son, Siddhartha, who was twenty-nine years old at the time, ventured out beyond the palace walls. There he saw for the first time in his life an old man, a sick man, a corpse, and, lastly, a renunciate with a very calm and peaceful face. Looking at the renunciate, the future Buddha knew that he had to follow that path. The next night, under cover of darkness, Siddhartha took one last look at his wife and infant son and then escaped from the palace in search of a cure for universal suffering.

For the next six years, Siddhartha led a severe ascetic life and studied various methods of meditation. Finally, almost at the brink of starvation, he accepted a bowl of rice from a young girl. At that moment he realized that extremism wasn't the answer. That night, at the age of thirty-five, Siddhartha sat down under a pipal tree and swore he wouldn't get up until he became fully enlightened. Going into deep meditation, he was tested by the forces of desire and death. He sat unwavering and at the crack of dawn, having overcome all negative forces, attained omniscience. For the next forty-five years, out of his great compassion for others, the Buddha traveled almost continuously, sharing with others what he had learned. He died at the age of eighty in 484 B.C.E.

His teachings became known as the Dharma. The Dharma explains that liberation can be achieved by anyone who realizes The Four Noble Truths. These are the following:

1. Suffering is universal and inevitable.

2. Desire is the immediate cause of suffering and ignorance the ultimate cause.

3. There is a way to get out of suffering.

4. The eightfold path of right view, right thought, right speech, right action, right livelihood, right effort, right mindfulness, and right contemplation is the way out of suffering.

JIVAKA KUMAR BHACCHA

During the Buddha's life, he was cared for by an Indian Ayurvedic doctor named Jivaka Kumar Bhaccha, who became one of the most famous physicians of his time. Years later, when Indian missionaries traveled throughout Asia, they brought with them the knowledge of this great doctor and surgeon. In Thailand, many Thais still consider him "The Father of Medicine."

His greatness as a doctor and surgeon was legendary. In *Tibetan Buddhist Medicine and Psychiatry* (Samuel Weiser, 1984), Terry Clifford writes: "His supreme skill as a physician was matched by his supreme devotion to Lord Buddha, whom he attended three times a day. The Buddha declared Jivaka to be chief among his lay followers. Because of his medical eminence, Jivaka was three times crowned in public as 'King of Doctors,' and is therefore known as the 'Thrice Crowned Physician' . . . He was an expert in pediatrics and

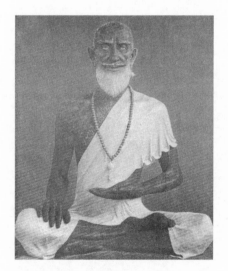

Dr. Jivaka Kumar Bhaccha

excelled in brain surgery. He successfully performed intricate abdominal operations."[3] He was also the personal physician of King Bimbisara of Magadha (a kingdom in what is now the state of Bihar in eastern India).

There are many different versions of Jivaka Kumar Bhaccha's birth and medical education. They all seem to agree, however, that he was born in Rajagriha (now Rajgir), which was the ancient capital of Magadha. Magadha rose to power under King Bimbisara around 540 B.C.E. According to Sanskrit-Tibetan and Chinese accounts, King Bimbisara was the father of Jivaka Kumar Bhaccha. Each version gives a different mother. In a Pali account, there is no mention of his father, just that he was born to a courtesan of Rajagriha. In any case, as Jivaka Kumar Bhaccha grew up, he decided that he wanted to study medicine. All accounts go on to say that he received advanced medical training in the city of Taxila (now in Pakistan) under Atreya, India's most renowned physician of the time.

To this day, Thai massage therapists show their veneration for Jivaka Kumar Bhaccha by performing *wai khru*. *Khru* means "teacher," and *wai khru* means "honoring the teacher." The words recited in the wai khru to Jivaka Kumar Bhaccha are mainly in Pali, with the remaining twenty percent in Sanskrit. Pali was the vernacular dialect of classical Sanskrit and was used to compose the sacred literature of Buddhism. It became the main literary language of the Buddhists. As Buddhism declined in India, Pali ceased to be used there. It remains, however, the main liturgical language in Thailand, Sri Lanka, and Myanmar. The fact that this wai khru is in Pali and Sanskrit, two ancient Indian languages, and not in Thai, and that it is in honor of an eminent Indian doctor are both indications that India played an important role in the development of Thai massage.

Many of the words in the wai khru are no longer recognizable, so the following English translation is only a rough idea of the prayer's meaning. Thai people pronounce Jivaka Kumar Bhaccha as *Shivago Komarpai*. Sometimes, such as in this wai khru, he is referred to simply as *Shivago*:

Homage to you, Shivago, who established the rules and precepts. I pray that kindness, wealth, medicine—everything comes to you. I pray to you who brings light to everyone just as the sun and moon do, who has perfect wisdom and who knows everything. We all love you

*who are without defilement, who are near to enlightenment—having
entered the stream three times. We all come to pray to you. I pray to
you. I pray to the Buddha. I pray, I pray that with your help all sick-
ness and disease will be released from whom I touch.*

The Pali-Sanskrit text of the wai khru appears in Chapter 9 on page 76.

SHARING OF MEDICAL THEORIES

So far India's early influence on Thai massage in the form of Ayurveda, yoga,
and Buddhism has been discussed, as well as China's influence, caused by the
two countries' proximity to each other, the large migrations of Chinese
people to Thailand throughout Thai history, the Silk Road, and the sea route.
Despite China's historical connection with Thailand, India, not China, is usually credited as the soul behind Thai massage. It therefore is important to ac-
knowledge that China also must have played a significant role. Furthermore,
due to the exchange of ideas between India and China since prehistoric
times, the divisions between them are not as distinct as one might think. Exchanges continued between these two great civilizations as Buddhism spread
from India along its northern and southern routes and the Silk Road. Therefore, to credit only one of these great countries' medical systems in Thailand's massage heritage is too simplistic. Over the centuries, both countries
must have significantly influenced the development of Thai massage.

Investigating the traditional energy systems that are part of Chinese,
Indian, and Thai medical understanding, many correspondences show up
between the Indian and Chinese systems, the Thai and Indian systems, and
the Thai and Chinese systems. As noted earlier, both the Indian and the
Thai system speak of 72,000 energy lines. Within that, each system has a
number of principal energy channels. In the Indian Ayurvedic model, there
are fourteen major nadis. In the Chinese traditional medical system,
there are fourteen principal meridians—twelve bilaterally symmetrical pairs
of cardinal conduits that interconnect through the fingers and toes, and
two of the eight odd conduits that fall on the midline of the body. In Thailand, some sources say that there are ten principal sen and others say that
there are fourteen.

The orifices are important in both the Thai and the Indian systems. According to Ayurvedic scholar David Frawley, "The best way to treat the nadis is to treat their different orifices or apertures, which are their main sites for reception and transmission of energy."[4]

Studies show that some exact and unmistakable correspondences exist between some of the Thai therapeutic points and some of the Chinese acupuncture points. Interestingly, all of the Chinese points that correspond with Thai points, except for one, are located on the meridians that have points on the trunk, legs, and head, namely the Stomach, Spleen, Urinary Bladder, Kidney, Gallbladder, Liver, Governing Vessel, and Conception Vessel meridians. The remaining meridians, namely the Heart, Small Intestine, Lung, Large Intestine, Pericardium, and Triple Heater, which have points on the trunk, arms, and head, do not have any corresponding points.

It is interesting to note that no corresponding points have been found between the Chinese meridians that travel on the arms and the Thai sen. This somehow seems to tie in with the Thai emphasis on leg work. Could it be that the Thais, when incorporating Chinese medicine, didn't bother taking their arm lines into account as they didn't feel they were important? Or did they create Sen Kalathari, which runs to all the fingers and toes as a "composite" meridian to correspond with the interconnecting that occurs through the fingers and toes in China's twelve main meridians? Further research will have to be done in order to explore why there are no corresponding points on the arms and to understand the Thai focus on the legs.

Returning to the similarities between India and China's traditional medical correspondences, one sees in fact that the two medical systems "possess an affinity for language, approach and methodology, with their emphasis on the life-force, the elements and qualities of nature. . . . Both systems speak of wind, fire and phlegm disorders and employ similar methodologies to treat them. Both systems classify food and herbs by taste, element and heating or cooling energy."[5] Furthermore, although Chinese medicine is usually associated with acupuncture, the system is predominantly herbal in nature. Likewise, Ayurveda, which is not commonly associated with acupuncture, has a whole system for treating special points known as marmas, which are positioned along the nadis (energy channels). In fact, one of the Vedas (sacred Hindu texts) is called the *Suchi Veda,* which literally means "the art of piercing with a needle." These similarities indicate much ancient cross-cultural sharing.

The five-element theory is a striking example that illustrates Thailand, China, and India's shared medical philosophies, their differences, and India's precedence over Thailand's traditional medical system. Both China's and India's traditional medical systems are based on five elements. In China, these are earth, water, fire, wood, and metal. In India, they are earth, water, fire, air, and ether. In Thailand, however, there are only four elements: earth, water, fire, and air. Although the first three elements are common to both China and India, air corresponds only to India's system, showing, in this case, the precedence of the Indian system over the Chinese in Thai massage.

Finally, it is interesting to look at the actual Thai term for massage, which is *Nuad Boran*. This literally means "ancient massage." It is not clear whether this means that Thai massage came from other ancient cultures or if it refers to an ancient indigenous Thai form.

More Recent History

In the thirteenth century, several principalities in Thailand joined together to form the Sukhothai Empire (1238–1378 C.E.), which the Thais consider their first true Thai kingdom. Sukhothai was taken over by the Ayuthaya kings, who ruled from 1350 to 1767 C.E. Thai medicine was codified sometime during the fifteen or sixteenth century. All important information was stored in the national archives in the capital of Ayuthaya. In the mid-sixteenth century, the Burmese invaded and took control of Ayuthaya. Fortunately, by the end of the century, the Thais had regained rule of their country. However, in 1765, the Burmese once again invaded Thailand and, according to Joe Cummings and Steve Martin's *Thailand* (Lonely Planet, 2001), "the capital fell after two years of fighting. This time the invaders destroyed everything sacred to the Thais, including manuscripts, temples and religious sculpture."[6]

Only two medical texts survived the Ayuthaya era: the *Pharmacopoeia of King Narai* and the *Scripture of Diseases*. Seven months after the fall of Ayuthaya, a young Thai general named General Phaya Taksin and his followers expelled the Burmese. General Taksin ruled from 1767 to 1772. After his death, General Chao Phraya Chakri—also known as King Rama I—

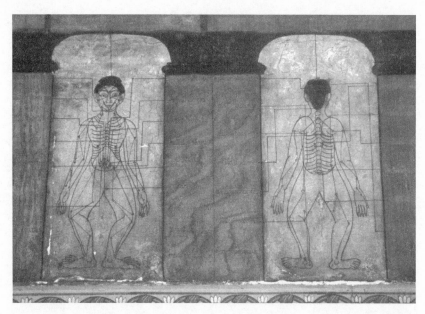

Plaques at Wat Pho

became the first king of the Chakri Dynasty, which has continued up to today's present King Rama IX.

King Rama III, who ruled from 1824 to 1851, played an important role in the preservation of Thai culture. He had information on religion, history, fine arts, and medicine collected from all over Thailand. This information was carefully studied. Next, in a brilliant move for posterity, King Rama III ordered the best of the information to be inscribed on the walls of Wat Phra Chetuphon. Today this encyclopedic work stands for all to see and study. Wat Phra Chetuphon, also known as Wat Pho, is one of the principal royal temples in Bangkok. It is also Bangkok's oldest temple and is famous for its Reclining Buddha statue.

King Rama III chose Wat Pho not only because it was a royal temple, but also because it was the earliest center for public education in Thailand.

Thai temples, which are known as *wats,* were and still often are the center of community life. They have been used for education, town meetings, social events, lodging, community storage, and health care, which was provided for by the monks. Today, maintaining that tradition, Wat Pho is the national center for preservation, research, treatment, and teaching of Thai massage in Thailand.

For Thai massage therapists, the medical inscriptions at Wat Pho are invaluable. Sixty stone plaques of the human body—thirty of the front and thirty of the back—have been inscribed there. On these figures, therapeutic points and energy pathways known as *sen* were engraved. Explanations were carved on the walls next to the plaques.

Thai massage is thriving in Thailand today, as more and more people realize the benefits of traditional medicine. The national government, through the Ministry of Health and Education, has recently begun a program to revive and pass on the traditional healing arts of Thailand. Due to Thai massage's increasing popularity, it is now also being practiced and taught in many other countries and has even found its way back to India.

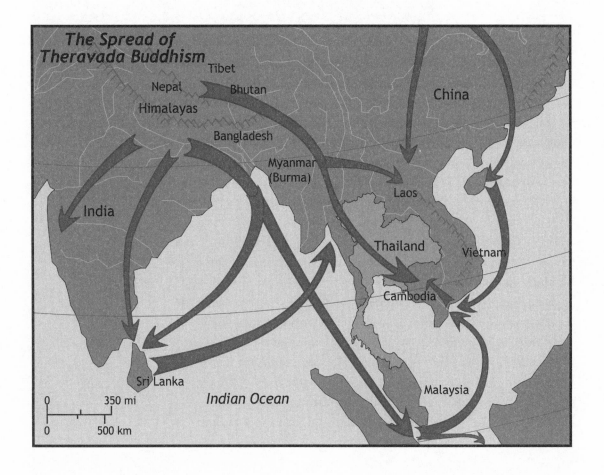

The Philosophical Foundations of Thai Massage

One of my masters told me that the more treatments you give, the more you will grow as a human being.

—James Mochizuki

What are the philosophical foundations upon which Thai massage rests? As mentioned before, Thai massage seems to have been influenced by Indian and Chinese traditional medical systems. Following is a more in-depth look at these systems, as well as the feminine/masculine principle, gravity, and the sen.

Ayurveda

Ayurveda is a holistic medical science that treats the whole person and takes into account the interconnectedness of the body, mind, and spirit. Due to this deep understanding, nothing is ever treated in isolation.

Ayurveda draws from a comprehensive background of medical knowledge, philosophy, religion, astrology, psychology, meditation, and astronomy. It treats imbalances through herbs, massage, marma puncture or acupressure, asana and pranayama practice, and diet. All of its medications come from natural substances, primarily herbs, which generally have no harmful effects when used properly.

Ayurveda is based on strong moral principles, which are believed to create a positive imprint on the mind thus enhancing health. The principles are to refrain from the following:

- Killing

- Stealing

- Lying

- Sexual misconduct

- Alcohol consumption

In Ayurveda, as noted earlier, there are five elements: ether, air, fire, water, and earth. Each person is composed of a combination of these five elements. Different combinations of these elements make up what are known as the three *doshas* (humors), which are vata, pitta, and kapha. Each dosha is a combination of two elements. Vata is a combination of the elements ether and air, pitta is a combination of the elements fire and water, and kapha is a combination of the elements water and earth.

Each person has a predominance of one of the three doshas and is therefore classified as a vata, pitta, or kapha type. David Frawley explains: "Yogic views of anatomy, physiology and psychology were originally formulated in terms of the doshas . . . an understanding of the ayurvedic constitutional types helps us adapt yoga practices according to individual requirements. The asanas, pranayama, and meditation practices appropriate for one doshic type may not be useful for another."[1]

Today, some Thai massage practitioners from the international community outside of Thailand are designing their treatment plans according to their clients' doshic makeup. They infer that since Thai massage has been historically linked with India's medical and religious traditions, including Ayurveda, this is a logical extension of Thai massage. Although this extension is possible, the consideration of doshas is not currently practiced in Thailand for traditional massage treatments and so it will not be discussed further in this book.

TRADITIONAL CHINESE MEDICINE

Traditional Chinese medicine, like Ayurveda, is a holistic medical science that treats the whole person. It uses herbs, acupuncture, and *tuina* (manual therapy). Its primary tenet is that everything is interconnected and that in order to live a healthy life, one must live in harmony with nature. It views wholeness as its beginning point.

Traditional Chinese medicine is based on the theory of *yin and yang, ki,* and the five elements. Yin and yang are seen as opposing yet complementary qualities. Within yin there is a seed of yang and within yang there is a seed of yin. Yang is traditionally regarded as the masculine quality and yin as the feminine. However, nothing in the universe is fully yin or yang, for all things are is relative to one another. For example, the moon, which is considered yin in relation to the sun, is yang in relation to the surrounding night sky. All life is dependent on the harmonious interaction of yin and yang. Traditional Chinese medicine aims at restoring a balance between these two principal forces of nature.

Ki, as mentioned earlier, is best explained as vital energy or force. It can be material or nonmaterial, matter or energy, depending on what form it assumes. The Chinese concept of ki ties in with the yin-yang theory, as ki arises out of the interaction of yin and yang. It is the most fundamental substance of the universe. Therapeutically speaking, ki, in its energetic form, is what flows through the body's energy channels.

The five-element theory developed later on in Chinese medical history and was then incorporated into the yin-yang theory. It postulates that all phenomena are one of five manifestations resulting from the transformation of ki. These five manifestations are known as the five elements and are symbolized as water, fire, wood, metal, and earth. Each of these elements relates to each of the others through the *creation cycle* or the *control cycle.* In traditional Chinese medicine, treatment consists of balancing the five elements through understanding these interrelationships.

There are twelve paired energy channels and eight unpaired energy channels in the body. These are usually known as meridians, and they can be treated through acupuncture, massage, or herbs. The result of treatment is a more balanced energy flow along the channels, which in turn influences organ function.

FEMININE/MASCULINE PRINCIPLES

The Thais believe that the left side of the body is the feminine side and the right side of the body is the masculine side. Therefore, in a traditional treatment, the left side of the body is treated first when working on a woman and the right side is treated first when working on a man. For example, if you are working on the feet one at a time and your client is a female, you would massage her left foot first and her right foot second.

I was unable to find more information on this in Thailand and so looked for answers further back in history. Fortunately, there is information in Ayurveda that deals with precisely this subject. In fact, just as in Thai massage, Dr. Frank Ros says that Ayurveda divides the body into "two opposite but interdependent halves, that is a left and a right half."[2] The left side is related to negative energy and is associated with the female; the right side is related to positive energy and is associated with the male.

The left side, the Ayurvedic texts say, is under the control of Ida Nadi, the energy line that originates at the left nostril, and the right side is under the control of Surya Nadi, which originates at the right nostril. Surya Nadi is also known as Pingala Nadi. Ida, the left nadi, dominates right-brain activity, which is feeling-oriented. Pingala, the right nadi, dominates left-brain activity, which is rationally oriented.

Interestingly, Thai massage also has two symmetrical energy lines, which run on the left and right sides of the body, are both connected with the nose, and have very similar names. The energy line on the left is known as Sen Ittha and the one on the right as Sen Pingkala. Notice the linguistic similarities: Ida and Ittha, Pingala and Pingkala. This further verifies the validity of looking for an explanation of the feminine/masculine principles within Ayurveda.

GRAVITY

The Thais noticed that the body is affected by gravity. In order to counter this, Thai massage was designed to work from the bottom up. This way, whatever is descending is encouraged to ascend. Therefore, the feet, being the lowest part of the body, are worked on first. The legs are worked on next and so forth up to the head, which is usually worked on in the last position. Inverted postures are also used in Thai massage to help counter gravity.

By working on the lower extremities first, energy is helped to move upward. For example, when the reflex points on the soles of the feet are pressed, the force should go all the way through the body to the head, which should move upward each time a reflex point is pressed. Similarly, when the legs are palmed or thumbed on, they are worked on from the bottom up.

Ideally, a person's energy will be evenly distributed throughout his or her body by the end of a Thai massage treatment. Ill health is the result of energy being stuck in one part of the body or another.

The concept of gravity also applies to the blood. Since the feet are at the lowest point in circulation, blood going from the feet toward the heart has the difficult task of going back up against gravity. Thai massage's inverted postures help the blood to move back toward the heart.

Thai massage therapists who start their treatments with the upper body—with the shoulders, for example—instead of starting at the feet are not following one of the most fundamental principles behind Thai massage. All traditional treatments in Thailand start with the feet and proceed up the body from there.

BUDDHISM

In Thailand, Buddhism is the official state religion and more than 95 percent of Thais are Buddhists. Most of the Thai people practice Theravada Buddhism. *Theravada,* which literally means "doctrine of the elders," is the older of the two forms of Buddhism, the other one being *Mahayana* Buddhism. Theravada Buddhists believe that their form more strictly adheres to the original teachings of the Buddha.

All Thai males are expected to be monks for some period of their lives. Usually, when they are young, they take vows for three months. If they wish to continue then or at a later time, it is highly esteemed and their families believe that they will earn great merit.

Very early in the morning, one can see these young orange-robed monks out on the streets with their large round begging bowls. Local people give them offerings of food and flowers. There are wats (temples) and monasteries throughout the country.

There also are nuns in Thailand, but their number is much smaller than that of the monks—10,000 as compared with 460,000. This is because nuns are not given the same respect as monks. Part of this has to do with the fact that merit is associated with the number of precepts one has taken. Thai nuns normally take eight vows, whereas Thai monks take 227, so the monks are held in much higher esteem. Furthermore, since nuns rarely perform ceremonies for laypeople, the laypeople feel less invested in making them offerings.

Theravada teaches that there are three principal aspects of existence. These are:

1. *Dukkha* (lack of satisfaction with existence).

2. *Anicca* (the lack of permanence for anything).

3. *Anatta* (the insubstantiality of reality).

The ultimate goal is the end of all grasping. When this is achieved, rebirth ceases as no attachment is left and one achieves *nibbana* (liberation). The consequences of attachment, the law of karma—which the Thais sum up as "Do good and good will follow; do bad and bad will follow"—and the acceptance of rebirth form the spiritual ideology of the Thai people. They devote much of their time to worship, making offerings at the temples, and feeding the monks in the hope of accumulating enough merit for a better rebirth or to achieve nibbana. The values of nonviolence, lovingkindness, and compassion are deeply instilled in the Thai people.

Traditional Thai medicine, which includes Thai massage, deeply reflects its Buddhist background. The following words from His Holiness The Dalai Lama describing Tibetan medicine could actually be used to describe Thai medicine:

> Tibetan medicine is deeply integrated with Buddhist practice and theory . . . The ideal doctor is one who combines sound medical understanding with strong realization of wisdom and compassion.[3]

His Holiness's words perfectly describe the spirit behind Thai medicine. It is regarded as a perfect spiritual practice, for it exemplifies the four divine states of mind, which are:

1. *Metta* (goodwill, lovingkindness).

2. *Karuna* (compassion, the desire to help others).

3. *Mudita* (sympathetic joy, gladness for the good fortune of others).

4. *Upekkha* (impartiality or equanimity).

This is why Thai medicine has held such an important position in the activities of the Thai temple.

THE SEN

In Thailand, energy lines are known as *sen*. What is a sen? There is no one word in the English language that can fully convey the meaning of this indigenous word. However, the following are words that can be associated with the sen:

- Conduits

- Channels

- Fibers

- Filaments

- Narrow ridge

- Line

- Sinew

- Tendon

The term *sen* can also appear as a prefix followed by a defining anatomical term such as:

- *Sennamlyang* = lymphatic (*namlyang* literally means "yellow fluid" and stands for lymph).

- *Senloohid* = blood vessel (*loohid* literally means "red color" or "blood").

- *Senloohiddeeng* = artery (*deeng* literally means "red").

- *Senloohiddam* = vein (*dam* literally means "black color," obviously indicating the darker color of venous blood).

Possibly the word *conduit* is the best word choice, as it encompasses all of the above meanings and implies the capacity of connecting as well as of conducting substances, including sensations, from one place to another.

As mentioned earlier, the Thai people believe that there are 72,000 energy lines, of which ten are considered the most important. Although it has been agreed that there are ten main sen, since they are invisible and do not have an anatomical base, descriptions of where they run, how they should be worked on, and what they do differ from school to school. Similarly, the therapeutic points used by different practitioners have not been nationally codified yet. In Thai massage, the main focus is on line work rather than on point work, as in acupuncture, for example.

Although the diagrams and descriptions at Wat Pho shed some light on the sen, the information is still incomplete and needs further research. What is apparent, though, is that the figures represent relationships between anatomical locations and the effects produced by treatment at those locations. In other words, the diagrams seem to represent therapeutic mechanisms.

From a Western point of view, the diagrams are not correct, anatomically speaking. This is not surprising, as traditional Thai medical training did not include dissection. I do not mean to imply, however, that the figures are merely fanciful. Are they possibly a stylized presentation of the body in a way we don't understand yet? They certainly, as has been said, "correspond respectively to the yin and yang surfaces of the trunk and limbs . . . as represented in Chinese anatomical drawings."[4]

In the treatment sequence described in Part Two of this book, only segments of the sen are worked on. On the legs, these segments are referred to as Inner and Outer Leg Lines 1, 2, 3, and 4; on the arms, they are referred to as Front and Back Arm Lines; and on the back, as the Back Line. This is for the convenience of Westerners; these names and numbers are not part of the traditional Thai way of teaching.

The following sections of this chapter contain descriptions and illustrations of the ten main sen, according to the perspective of Pichest Boonthumme. All of them start at or near the navel and are connected with various orifices in the body, such as the eyes or ears. Since the pathways are invisible, and since many of them travel deep within the body, they are very difficult to put down on paper. The illustrations are therefore only rough maps of an invisible landscape. Precise knowledge of where the sen run and their effects is not necessary when doing a basic treatment, for simply by doing a session the sen are worked on anyway. Even Thai massage practitioners with years of experience have difficulty feeling the sen lines, which are for the most part intangible. The sens' lack of precise anatomical location, combined with their lack of solidity, helps to explain why there is so much controversy in Thailand about their location and effect. The main thing to remember is to be open to the concept of energy and to recognize that more affects the body than can be seen with the naked eye. It is not necessary to memorize the information on the sen in order to give a good Thai massage, although it is good to be familiar with it. Just be open to the concept of energy lines, and over time a feeling for them will develop.

In the illustrations, an X has been used to mark the beginning of each sen. Solid lines indicate sen pathways that run on or just near to the surface of the body. Broken lines indicate sen pathways that run deep within the body.

1. Sen Sumana

Sen Sumana is connected with the blood and can be felt at various pulses on the body. It runs along the midline of the front and back of the body as well as in the arms and legs. While Sen Sumana is circling the midline of the body, it is also simultaneously circling in the arms and legs. Since it is very hard to know exactly where Sen Sumana runs in the body, for the sake of simplicity only the most prominent aspect of it has been illustrated. This aspect begins two onkkulee (an onkkulee is the length of one bone in the index finger) above the navel on the midline of the body. From there, it travels up the chest inside the neck through the jaw to the bottom of the tongue.

Notes

Sen Sumana is connected with the mouth. Its actual literal translation is "origin at the tongue." Some theories state that it begins at the tongue and others that it begins above the navel. Its orifice is the mouth.

Sen Sumana's location and function is similar to the Ren Mai Channel (Conception Vessel) and the Du Mai Channel (Governing Vessel) in Chinese acupuncture.

Sen Sumana's location and function is also similar to Sushumna Nadi in Indian yoga. Both channels run on the midline of the body and involve the spinal canal. Both are considered the most important channels of their system. Sushumna Nadi has the nature of fire and is activated by the kundalini—latent spiritual energy situated at the base of the spine that can be awakened and made to go up the spinal column to the brain. When the kundalini is fully awakened, one becomes enlightened. The chakras (spinning energy centers that transform psychophysical energy into spiritual energy) are located in the spinal cord. Notice also the linguistic similarity of the words *Sumana* and *Sushumna*. This again seems to indicate that Thai massage originated in India or that India played a significant role in the development of Thai massage.

Any problem that shows up in Sen Sumana will eventually show up in other sen if the condition becomes chronic.

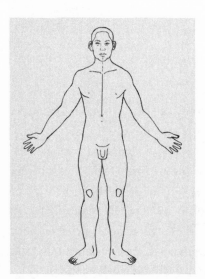

Figure 5.1: Sen Sumana

Treatment Applications

Work on Sen Sumana is good for improving general energy. Asthma; bronchitis; chest pain; throat, tongue, and speech problems; lower back problems; numbness; stiffness; and paralysis are a few of the conditions that benefit from working on Sen Sumana.

Stopping and then releasing the blood at the pulses, which, as mentioned before, is connected with Sen Sumana, brings fresh blood carrying oxygen and nutrients to the area and helps to remove waste products and toxins. The pulses that are the most easy to feel are the popliteal pulse (felt over the popliteal artery behind the knee), the posterior tibial pulse (felt over the posterior tibial artery on the medial [inner] side of the ankle), the femoral pulse (felt over the femoral artery at the inguinal crease [where the leg joins the trunk]), the brachial pulse (felt over the brachial artery in the armpit), and the radial pulse (felt over the radial artery on the wrist). Blood stopping is most often done at the femoral pulse, but sometimes it is done at the brachial pulse.

If you are working on someone who has high blood pressure, do not stop the blood nor work on Sen Sumana. If a person has low blood pressure, stop the blood for half the amount of time you normally would.

2. Sen Ittha and 3. Sen Pingkhala

These two sen travel the same route, although on the opposite sides of the body. Sen Ittha travels on the left and Sen Pingkhala travels on the right. Following is a description of Sen Ittha's pathway.

Sen Ittha starts two onkkulee to the left of the navel. From there, it runs up the torso to just above the level of the left nipple, where it turns left and goes to the left armpit. At the armpit, it meets a branch that starts at the back of the left side of the neck, just above the seventh cervical (neck) vertebra and then passes many sensitive points on the shoulder blade on its route to the armpit. The two lines then travel from the armpit to the end of the left little finger as parallel streams on the front and back surfaces on the medial side of the left arm and hand. They then retrace themselves up the hand and arm along the same route they descended. The front line, after returning to the armpit, runs up across the left pectoral muscle, under the left collarbone, up the left side of the neck and face to the side of the left nostril. From there, it goes up over the left side of the head and then down the left side of the neck beside the cervical spine. On its descent, as mentioned before, it branches out to the left armpit. The main trunk continues down beside the spine to the middle of the left buttock and then passes through the body, emerging at the starting place two onkkulee to the left of the navel. From there, it runs down the left side of the abdomen to the left femoral pulse. From the femoral pulse, it travels down the left front thigh to the left knee, which it passes through, coming out on the back of the left lower leg. It runs down the left lower leg to the left ankle and then along the outer side of the left foot to the end of the left little toe. The line then retraces itself up the foot, lower leg, and thigh to the femoral pulse. At the femoral pulse, there is a pathway that connects Sen Ittha with Sen Pingkhala. From the femoral pulse, Sen Ittha goes back to its original starting place two onkkulee to the left of the navel.

Notes

Sen Ittha and Sen Pingkhala are connected with the nose. Their orifices are the left and right nostril, respectively.

Ittha literally means "moon left side" and *pingkhala* literally means "the sun progresses right."

Sen Ittha and Sen Pingkhala correspond to Ida and Pingala Nadi, which are the two second most important nadis in yoga. There is also a linguistic similarity between the words *Ittha* and *Ida, Pingkhala* and *Pingala,* and they share the concept of dividing the body into left and right halves, with the left half being under the control of Sen Ittha in the Thai system and Ida Nadi in the Indian system, and the right half being under the control of Sen Pingkhala in the Thai system and Pingala Nadi in the Indian system. Both systems have the nostrils as their orifice. Ida Nadi is said to have lunar energy, which ties in with the Thai translation of *Ittha*—"moon, left side." Similarly, Pingala Nadi has solar energy, which ties in with the Thai translation of Pingkhala—"the sun progresses right." Normally, the breath flows in one of these two channels, alternating every few hours according to various environmental, constitutional, and time factors. The breath in the right nostril is said to be hot. It is therefore called the sun breath, and the right

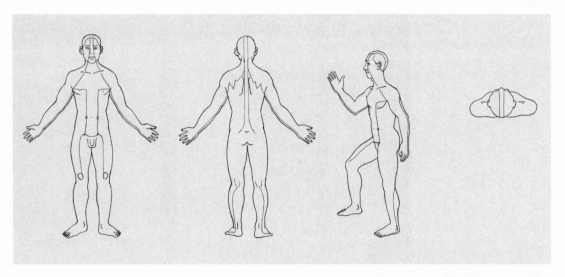

Figure 5.2: Sen Ittha and Sen Pingkhala

nadi is referred to as *pingala* ("of the color of fire"). Similarly, the breath in the left nostril is said to be cool. It is therefore called the moon breath and is referred to as *ida*. Ida and Pingala intersect each other along the Sushumna at various places like a series of figure eights one on top of the other. These junctions are called chakras. There are seven chakras in the body.

Sen Ittha and Sen Pingkhala form the medial (inner-side) half of Sen Sumana in the forearm and hands.

Problems that show up in Sen Ittha and Sen Pingkhala are manifestations of chronic conditions that, in the acute stage, showed up in Sen Sumana.

Treatment Applications

Problems with internal and external rotation of the arms; muscular and joint problems in the elbows, neck, shoulders, back, and knees; abdominal problems; headaches; colds; coughs; and sinus problems are a few of the conditions that benefit from working on Sen Ittha and Sen Pingkhala.

4. Sen Kalathari

Sen Kalathari starts at the navel, where it divides into four lines like an X that travels symmetrically on both sides of the body. The top two lines travel up

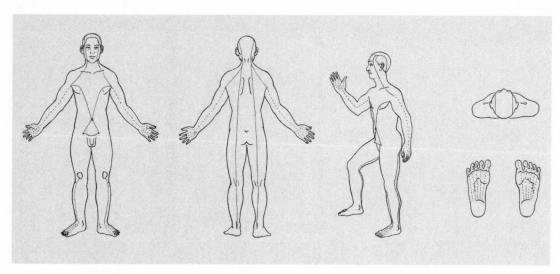

Figure 5.3: Sen Kalathari

to the armpits, passing above the nipples on the way. From there, they travel inside the middle of the arms to the wrists. At the wrists, Sen Kalathari splits into five branches, with each branch running to the tip of a finger. They then retrace themselves up the hands and arms, to the collarbones which they run under, up the sides of the front of the neck and face, over the temples to the end of the eyebrows. From there, they run up over the sides of the head and then down the back sides of the neck. Just below the neck, they branch off to the armpits, where they merge with the aforementioned lines traveling inside the middle of the arms. The main trunks continue down the back to the ischial tuberosities (the bones at the bottom of the pelvis that bear the body's weight when you are sitting down—commonly known as the "sit bones"). From there, they go down the backs of the thighs to the backs of the knees. From the backs of the knees, they travel down the middle of the backs of the calves to the feet. At the feet, Sen Kalathari splits into five branches, with each branch running to the tip of a toe. Sen Kalathari then retraces itself up the feet and then travels up the fronts of the lower legs to the knees. It goes through the knee joints and then travels up the backs of the thighs to the ischial tuberosities. From there, it goes through the legs to the femoral pulses in the inner upper thighs, where there is a pathway from one femoral pulse to the other, connecting the right and left lines. From the femoral pulses, Sen Kalathari returns to its starting place at the navel.

Notes

Sen Kalathari is connected with the navel. The orifice is the navel.

The literal translation of *kalathari* is "the twenty fingers and toes."

Sen Kalathari's connection with the fingers and toes is similar to the peripheral linkage of the fingers and toes in the Chinese meridian system.

Treatment Applications

Foot, hand, arm, and leg numbness, pain, and paralysis; knee problems; stiffness of the neck; shoulder problems; and various mental disorders are a few of the conditions that benefit from working on Sen Kalathari.

5. Sen Sahatsarangsi and 6. Sen Thawari

These two sen lines travel the same route, although on the opposite sides of the body. Sen Sahatsarangsi travels on the left. Sen Thawari travels on the right. Following is a description of Sen Sahatsarangsi's pathway.

Sen Sahatsarangsi starts at the waistline, four onkkulee to the left side of the navel. From there, it runs up the chest to the left nipple and then continues up to the left collarbone, runs under the collarbone, and proceeds to the left carotid pulse, which is felt in the neck to the side of the trachea (windpipe). At the pulse, it splits into two branches. One branch goes down to the hollow just above the jugular notch (the notch at the top of the sternum), where it connects with Sen Thawari. The other branch goes under the collarbone to the left arm. It proceeds down the front side of the arm to the hand, where it runs to the tip of the thumb. It then retraces itself up the hand and arm, under the collarbone, up the neck, inside the head to the inner corner of the left eye. From there, it runs over the head, down the neck, to several sensitive points on the shoulder blade, down the back and waist to the buttock, where it passes three sensitive points. From the buttock, it goes down the back of the thigh and lower leg. It circles under the foot just above the heel and then travels up the inner side of the lower leg and thigh to the

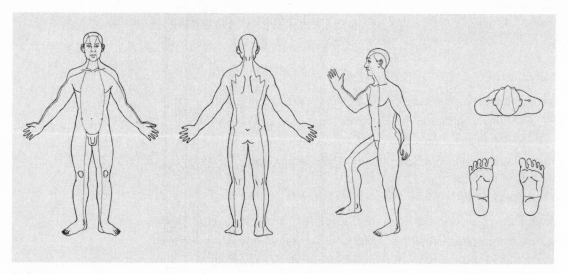

Figure 5.4: Sen Sahatsarangsi and Sen Thawari

femoral pulse. Here, there is a pathway between the two femoral pulses that connects Sen Sahatsarangsi with Sen Thawari. From the femoral pulse, it goes back to its original starting point four onkkulee to the left of the navel.

Notes

Sen Sahatsarangsi and Sen Thawari are connected with the eyes. *Sahatsarangsi* literally means "origin at the left eye," and *thawari* literally means "origin at the right eye." Their orifices are the left eye and right eye, respectively.

Sen Sahatsarangsi and Sen Thawari form the lateral side of Sen Sumana in the forearm and hands.

Sen Sahatsarangsi and Sen Thawari are connected with Sen Ittha and Sen Pingkhala and have similar pathways.

Treatment Applications

Muscular problems, joint problems, facial paralysis, and gastrointestinal diseases are a few of the conditions that benefit from working on Sen Sahatsarangsi and Sen Thawari. As Sen Sahatsarangsi and Sen Thawari are connected with Sen Ittha and Sen Pingkhala, any problems that benefit from treatment on Sen Ittha and Sen Pingkhala will also benefit here and vice versa.

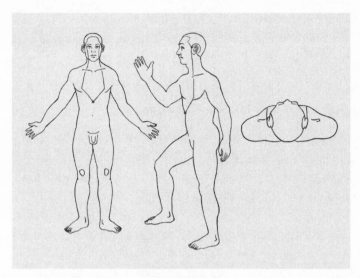

Figure 5.5: Sen Lawusang and Sen Ulangka

7. Sen Lawusang and 8. Sen Ulangka

These two sen lines travel the same route but on the opposite sides of the body. Sen Lawusang travels on the left and Sen Ulangka travels on the right. Following is a description of Sen Lawusang's pathway.

Sen Lawusang begins four onkkulee up from the navel, just under the xiphoid process (the lowest portion of the sternum). From there, it goes up to the left nipple. It continues up the chest, under the collarbone, up the neck and jaw to the ear, which it runs around. It then returns to its starting place via the same route.

Notes

Sen Lawusang and Sen Ulangka are connected with the ears. Sen Lawusang is also called *Sen Chanthaphusang,* which literally means "origin at the left ear." Sen Ulangka is also called *Sen Rucham,* which literally means "origin at the right ear." Their orifices are the left ear and the right ear, respectively.

Treatment Applications

Deafness, ear diseases, cough, toothache, sore throat, jaw problems, facial paralysis, and chest pain are some of the conditions that benefit from working on Sen Lawusang and Sen Ulangka. Being at high altitude, such as when flying in an airplane, affects the ears and Sen Lawusang and Sen Ulangka. Chewing gum can help then.

9. Sen Nanthakrawat and 10. Sen Khitchanna

Sen Nanthakrawat starts at the navel. In women, it runs via Sen Sikhini to the urethra. In men, it runs via Sen Sukhumung to the anus.

Sen Khitchanna starts at the navel. In women, it runs via Sen Khitcha to the vagina. In men, it runs via Sen Pitakun to the penis.

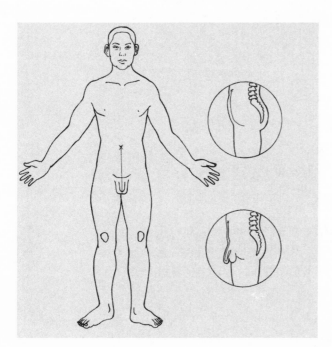

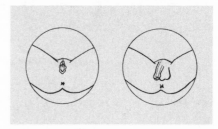

5.6: Sen Nanthakrawat

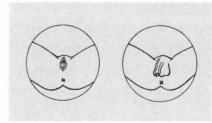

5.7: Sen Khitchanna

Notes

Sen Sikhini is connected with the urethra. *Sikhini* means "urinary passage." Its orifice is the urethra. Sen Sukhumung is connected with the anus. *Sukhumung* means "origin at the anus." Its orifice is the anus. The routes of Sen Khitchanna and Sen Nanthakrawat overlap.

There is much confusion about these two sen due to problems with translation from the original Sanskrit and Pali to Thai. Different books have different translations and different drawings to illustrate these two sen. Further research is necessary for greater clarification on their pathways.

Treatment Applications

Frequent urination, retention of urine, prostate problems, kidney stones and other kidney problems, female infertility, irregular menstruation, uterine bleeding, and impotence are some of the conditions that benefit from working on Sen Nanthakrawat and Sen Khitchanna.

CHAPTER

6

EMOTIONS AND THE BODY

Great compassion and wisdom are the chief qualities of the Buddha. Even in worldly terms, the more intelligent and knowledgeable a person is, the more the person commands respect. Similarly, the more compassionate, kind and gentle a person, the more he or she should be respected. So if you are able to develop that intelligence and altruism to their fullest extent, then you are truly admirable and deserve to be respected.

—HIS HOLINESS THE DALAI LAMA

Although Thai massage does not traditionally address the psychological aspect of bodywork, massage by its very nature does, and Thai massage is certainly no exception. Furthermore, since Thai massage not only uses massage, but also uses movement, it can have an even greater psychological impact. Through heightened awareness of holding patterns, movement can be a powerful tool to connect with subconscious memories held within the body. Finally, the intimate nature of the dance done between the therapist and the recipient in Thai massage may bring up emotions.

The body stores memories of all of life's experiences. Nothing, no matter how inconsequential, painful, or enjoyable, is censored. Even years later, the body will remember in every cell, nerve, muscle, and bone all that happened, unless some method of clearing has been used to release the body-mind-spirit of these memories.

Joan Borysenko, Ph.D., speaks of this when she says, "The body stores emotions rather than words. In order to heal, the emotions held within the body need to be acknowledged and then released. Touch is one of the best ways of facilitating this alchemical transmutation of wounds into wisdom."[1]

Touch by itself, however, doesn't usually have this evocative power. It is the quality of the touch that makes all the difference. Ilana Rubenfeld, author of *The Listening Hand* (Bantam Doubleday Dell, 2001), so aptly calls this quality "listening touch." This kind of touch conveys real attentiveness, real care about the person you are with. It requires being fully present in the moment. Such compassionate focus is felt by the recipient, who then feels safe enough to reconnect with experiences from the past.

Different parts of the body store different feelings and different memories. Some areas are more vulnerable than others. Likewise, different movements elicit different responses. Since Thai massage uses such a great variety of movements, the whole body is explored. A client of mine once said to me, "Wow, this really is detective work you are doing." She went on to say that until she got the massage with me she had never connected her current pain with an accident she had had years ago, which her conscious mind had totally forgotten about.

The body gives countless clues, and it is up to the practitioner to bring these to the awareness of the person being treated and then to help him or her with processing whatever comes up. Many people aren't even aware of their holding patterns, which over a long period of time can come to feel natural. One can point out the pattern verbally, but this usually has little effect. The person must become aware of the pattern on a kinesthetic level. This is where touch plays such an important role, as it enables the individual to feel the pattern inside his or her own body. Once the connection has been made physically, emotional healing can begin.

Although Thai massage addresses the whole body, it focuses a lot of its attention on the legs. Since the legs are connected with the pelvis, work on the legs has a ripple effect on the pelvis, which in turn can affect the sexual organs housed there. Let's take a look at the simple movement of externally rotating the legs. For someone who has been sexually traumatized, the opening movement of the legs can bring up tremendous feelings of fear, pain, and/or anxiety. The person may not even remember the painful incident, especially if it happened in early childhood, but the body has recorded it and remembers. The body-mind will unconsciously try to protect itself by resisting the rotation. There will be resistance as long as the body-mind tries to protect itself. This is where the practitioner's perception and skill come in. First, he or she must notice the holding pattern. Then the practitioner has to gently help the recipient to notice it. Finally, he or she needs to be able to guide the person to the inner meaning of it. In the process, what was before hidden is revealed. Healing can then occur as the trauma is released from the body-mind-spirit. When the work reaches this level, it is truly a healing modality, for it brings transformation at the deepest level.

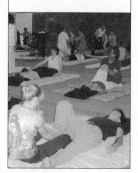

Thai Massage Workshop at the
Omega Institute

THE PRACTICE

Massage is not technique, but spirit . . . Your best teacher is your client's body . . . Learn to see the body through your fingertips; the fingertips are the eyes of the therapist. Learn to read the contours, tightness and temperature differences of the client's body. Listen to the body for the body will tell you what needs to be done.

—JAMES MOCHIZUKI

Body Mechanics Used in Thai Massage

*We should take this good heart, this altruism, as the very basis
and internal structure of our practice, and should direct whatever
virtuous activities we do towards its increase higher and higher.*

—His Holiness The Dalai Lama

T hai massage should be done in a rhythmical, relaxed manner at a
moderate pace. A dancelike quality should prevail, with fluidity and
grace permeating the session. Continuity should be maintained and each
transition should link prior and future movements together effortlessly.

It is most important to be *present* as you work—present to your own
body and feelings and your client's body and feelings. They are both equally
important. Notice how you use your body. The better your body mechanics
and the more comfortable you are, the more profound your session will be.
Likewise, notice your breath. Is it flowing or are you holding it? And where
is your mind? Are you truly present or are you thinking about something
else? Give the person you are treating your full attention. Don't have part of
your mind wandering off somewhere else. Do your work as a meditation
practice in the art of being present. If you find your mind wandering, come
back to the present moment. Thich Nhat Hanh, revered Buddhist teacher,
has a beautiful chant for this:

In . . . out . . . deep . . . slow.
Calm . . . ease . . . smile . . . release.
Present moment . . . wonderful moment.

Since Thai massage is very physical, good body mechanics are essential. With good body mechanics, you can do your work more effectively and with less effort. Your weight should be distributed between whatever parts of your body you are working with, such as your hands, elbows, knees, and/ or feet. Your back should be a little bit concave and your shoulders relaxed. When applying pressure, keep your arms or legs straight so that leaning power rather than muscular force is primarily used.

The position of the person you are treating is equally important. Since performing Thai massage involves moving the receiver from posture to posture, make sure to keep him or her properly aligned. This will make your work easier and your partner more comfortable.

Touch should be used first as a means of gathering information—that is, as diagnosis—and therapeutically. With this approach, the initial contact within a technique should be lighter than the later contact, as at first you are just trying to pick up information and then you are trying to effect change. In general, pressure should build from soft, to medium, to strong for each technique.

Perpendicular leaning pressure should be used for applying weight, and progressively stronger stretches should be used for stretching. You should rock from side to side or from front to back as you work so as to slowly shift your weight.

It is also important, as a general rule, to have your "center"—your abdominal area—facing the recipient and to work from this center. The Japanese call this area the *hara*. The hara is focused on in many Asian meditation and martial art practices to cultivate internal power. Although Thai massage doesn't speak about this, working from this center will improve the quality of your work. Pichest Boonthumme certainly works from this area. He is a slightly built man, but because he works from this center, he can transmit tremendous force.

Even with optimum body mechanics and with hara awareness, there are limitations. If the person you are working on is much bigger and/or heavier than you are, be careful when doing the lifts. There are some movements that you may have to avoid altogether. When you do a lift, remember to bend your knees rather than your back. Otherwise, you will risk injuring it. Also, if someone's body is very stiff, the work will be more difficult. This too must be taken into account.

Pressure-Applying Techniques

Many parts of the body can be used for applying pressure—the palm, thumb, elbow, feet, and knees. Most of the terms for specific techniques are self-explanatory—such as knee pressing, which literally means pressing with the knee—but some are not as obvious. Following are descriptions and photographs illustrating the less obvious ones.

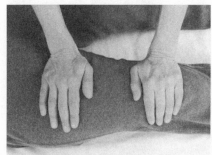

Palming. The palms of the hands "walk," one after the other.

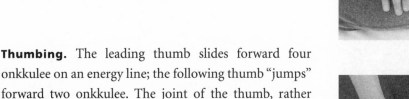

Thumbing. The leading thumb slides forward four onkkulee on an energy line; the following thumb "jumps" forward two onkkulee. The joint of the thumb, rather than the tip or the pad, is used to apply pressure.

Two kinds of thumbing are used when working the energy lines. The first is thumbing with the thumbs horizontally placed in the energy line's pathway. The second is thumbing with the thumbs vertically placed crossing the energy line's pathway.

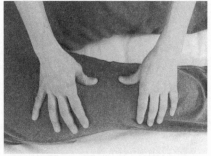

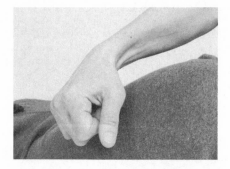

Tapotement (pronounced tah-pote-mahn). A loose fist is used to hit the area being treated with medium force.

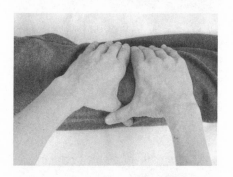

Chopping. The two palms are joined together with the fingers spread open. The heels of the hands are kept separate. The elbows are brought forward. The chopping movement comes from the rotation of the wrist and from the fingers coming together. Contact is made with the little fingers and the ends of the ring fingers. The chopping is done with medium force.

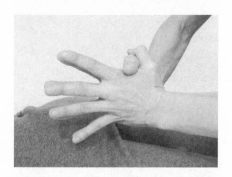

Crossed Thumbs. One thumb is crossed over the other and medium to strong pressure is applied through the thumb joints. Grip with your fingers as you press through your thumbs.

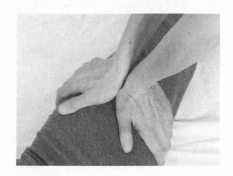

Butterfly Hands. The heels of the hands are near each other and the fingers face away. In some modified postures, the heels of the hands are a little further away from each other. The pressure comes mainly through the heels of the hands. Apply medium to strong force.

POSITIONS

In addition to employing specific techniques to apply pressure, the practitioner uses a number of body postures to administer Thai massage. Following are descriptions and photographs illustrating the main positions used by the practitioner.

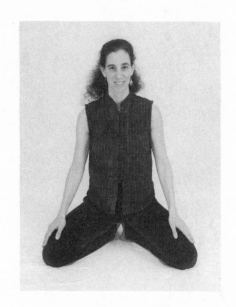

Kneeling. The knees and feet are together or the knees are spread open. The feet are flat or up on the toes.

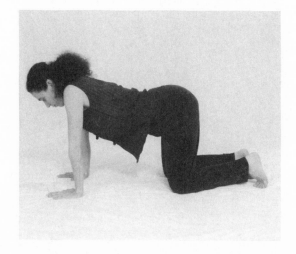

Crawling. The hands are below the shoulders, the knees below the hips, the arms straight, the feet up on the toes, and the back concave.

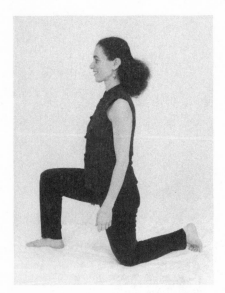

Half Lunge. The knee of one leg is below that hip on the floor. The knee of the other leg is up, with the thigh parallel to the floor and the foot below the knee.

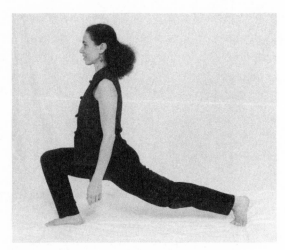

Full Lunge. This is the same as the half lunge but the leg that had the knee down is now up and stretched out.

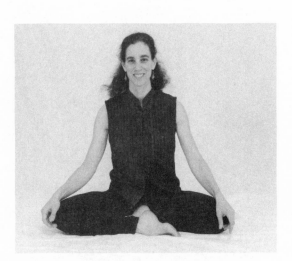

Sitting. The buttocks, legs, and feet are on the floor.

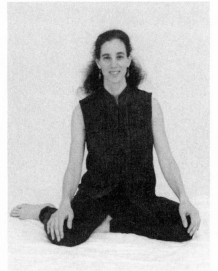

Thai Sitting. Both legs are bent to the side.

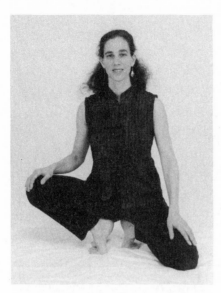

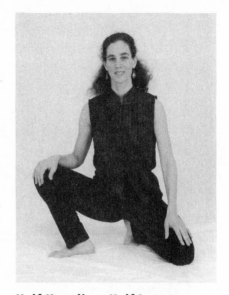

Half Kneeling, Half Squatting.
One leg is kneeling; the other
is squatting.

Half Kneeling, Half Lunge.
One leg is kneeling; the other is in
a half-lunge position.

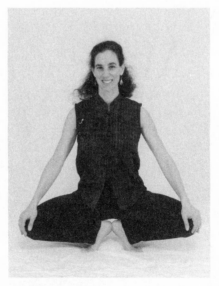

Squatting. The toes are
squatted on.

8

THE SESSION: PREPARATION, EFFECTS, AND CLOSURE

With genuine love and compassion, another person's appearance or behavior has no effect on your attitude. Real compassion comes from seeing the other's suffering. You feel a sense of responsibility, and you want to do something for him or her.

—HIS HOLINESS THE DALAI LAMA

Many factors contribute to making a session a truly healing experience. How you prepare, open, go through, and close a treatment are all equally important aspects. They determine the effectiveness of the session.

PREPARATION

Preparation for the session plays a very important role in its success. Most important of all is who you are—your essential being. This essential self will shine through all you do to the receiver. If you bring sincerity, enthusiasm, presence, and experience with you to the session, it is bound to be helpful. The more you study, and give and receive sessions, the more effective your treatments will be. Knowledge of the receiver's health issues before the session begins will enable you to plan your session better. Also, it is good to clear the space energetically before the treatment. This can be done through prayer, meditation, visualization, and/or the burning of sage and incense, as well as by beautifying the space you will be working in prior to the session.

TRAINING AND PRACTICE

Good training and lots of practice are key elements in one's development as a Thai massage therapist. Satish Kumar, keynote speaker at the Omega Institute's environmental conferences and chief editor of *Resurgence* magazine, spoke about practice. He said that, "In the Western languages, English especially, the word practice comes after theory, but in the Indian languages, particularly Sanskrit, it is the other way around—practice and then theory." In Thai massage this holds true, for no matter how much theory you learn or how often you watch a great master give treatments, it is really your own experience—what you gather directly—that will help you the most. James Mochizuki, Anma therapist and teacher, reinforces this concept when he tells his students, "Your best teacher is your client's body." Pichest Boon-thumme feels the same way and emphasizes practice. When students ask him for a certificate, he always laughs with a mixture of amusement and concern and says, "Later, after you have completed a thousand treatments and recorded every one." My shiatsu teacher in Japan, Oyamada sensei, also always said to practice and to feel. To every question I once asked him, through an expensive translator I had hired, he just said, "Feel." For months after that, while I was giving treatments, I heard his voice saying to me, "Just feel, just feel," and I would see him in front of my mind's eye carefully feeling as he worked, even after decades of experience. For him it was always a new moment—a new experience.

Experiential learning is an exciting process, for there is always more to learn, deeper levels of feelings to touch upon, and greater appreciation of the miracle of healing to tap into. So practice as much as you can. Once you feel comfortable with the techniques in this book, be creative and try new things. Take note of what you experience during each session so that you can grow from them. Most importantly, realize the preciousness of time shared with another human being and the grace of interacting in such a profound way.

Health Interview

Before giving a session, make sure to ask the recipient about his or her health. Even if the person is someone you already know well, it is important to check in again. If they are new to you, this is even more essential. Ask questions such as whether he or she has pain or sensitivity anywhere. Does he have any acute condition or chronic desease? How is his blood pressure? Has she had any accidents? Does she have varicose veins or any other circulatory problems? Is she pregnant or menstruating?

When hearing about the recipient's health concerns, it is important to remember that illness comes as a messenger of where imbalance has occurred. It is a direct reminder that we can't avoid, and in that sense it is a blessing in disguise, helping us to readjust our balance and come back to a more peaceful connection with life.

During the health interview, if the person you will be working on has never had a Thai massage before, give him or her a simple explanation of what Thai massage is. Also ask the person to let you know if anything feels uncomfortable during the treatment or if something feels good and should be repeated. Ask the recipient how your pressure feels and if the stretching is okay. As everyone is different, feedback is very useful. For example, some people like getting their toes cracked and others don't. Many people, however, are shy about giving feedback and suffer through a treatment not really getting what they need or want. This is why it is important to really tune in to the recipient and to take note of any clues that are given.

Treatment

I recommend that before starting the treatment you check the recipient's spine, although this is not traditionally done in Thailand. Look at it and then slide your palm down his or her back, over the spine. Repeat this as he or she slowly bends over and then comes back up. Feeling the spine like this will immediately give you information about the spine's condition, which has a tremendous impact on the rest of the body. Does the person have kyphosis (an exaggerated convex, or outward, curvature of the thoracic spine) or lordosis (an exaggerated concave, or inward, curvature of the lumbar spine) or scoliosis (side-to-side curvature of the spine)? By checking out the spine and before you give a treatment, you will understand better why the body is as it is.

Based on the health interview, you will have some idea of what needs to be done during the session. For example, if the person you will be working on is pregnant, you should do most of the treatment with her in the side-lying and seated position. Based on the recipient's condition and the time you have available, you can decide which parts of the routine you would like to use. Of course, even with a plan, as you actually do the work, you will learn more from the recipient's body, which will further determine which techniques you work with and which ones you delete. It is important beforehand to know the contraindications that follow.

CONTRAINDICATIONS

Because Thai massage involves so much movement of the body, it is important to not overstretch or overtwist anyone, as the potential for injury is there. Therefore, keep tuned! In addition, there are the standard contraindications that apply to all bodywork, as well as a few that are specific to this style of bodywork. Do not give Thai massage if:

- Either you or the other person is under the influence of drugs or alcohol.

- The person has an acute or chronic disease (unless you have the permission of a doctor).

- The person has cancer, pus formations, tuberculosis, or cystic (fluid-containing) tumors, as the massage might aid the proliferation of tumorous tissues or disperse infective material through the tissues.

- The person has a contagious illness.

- The person has a bone disease (unless you have the permission of a doctor).

- The person has a bone fracture or joint dislocation.

- The person is on cortisone treatment (which weakens the bone structure) or any other medication (unless you know the reason and have the permission of a doctor).

- The person has a high fever (unless you know and understand what is causing it and have a doctor's approval).

In addition, there are certain conditions that limit the techniques you should use, including the following:

- If the recipient is pregnant, do not give any stomach massage. After the third month of pregnancy, do not do anything that will cause pressure on the stomach. Also avoid pressing on the point on Inside Leg Line 2 one hand's breadth up from the inner protrusion of the anklebone. This point is known as SP 6 in acupuncture and shiatsu, and can cause contractions of the uterus.

- If the person has any open wounds, infections, blisters, and/or pimples, avoid those areas.

- If the person has any kind of circulatory problem, such as heart disease, high blood pressure, varicose veins, or diabetic neuropathy, do not use the blood-stopping technique.

- If the person has high blood pressure, do not do inverted postures.

The Setting

As mentioned earlier, a pleasant, clean, and peaceful environment helps to create the right atmosphere even before the massage begins. Beautiful and/or sacred paintings, photographs, and other objects enhance positive vibrations, as do plants and fresh flowers, incense, and candles. Use natural or soft artificial lighting. Background music can enhance the atmosphere. The temperature should be warm and comfortable. Good ventilation is a must.

The Mat

Thai massage is not done on a massage table, but on a mat on the floor. It's best to use a two- to four-inch-thick futon mat made of cotton or cotton with foam in the middle, plus a small pillow. The firmness of the futon is essential, for if it is too soft, it will absorb your pressure and make it difficult for you to keep your balance. Cover the futon with a sheet and have a blanket and bolsters nearby, in case your partner gets cold or needs support.

I highly recommend the futon mats sold by Thai Yoga Healing Arts. They are 100-percent cotton futon mats that roll up and tie with two straps. They are very comfortable as well as portable, and are available in natural and a variety of colors. For further information, see the Resources section at the back of the book.

If you don't have a carpet on your floor, I have found that the type of padding that is used under carpets works well as extra padding under the futon. You can cut a pad to fit exactly under your futon mat. Carpet padding is inexpensive, lightweight, and very portable.

Clothing

Thai massage is a "clothes-on" modality. Both the person giving the massage and the person receiving it should dress in light, loose comfortable clothes that allow for easy movement, as there is a lot of stretching, assisted yoga, and joint mobilization involved. Women should wear pants or shorts—skirts or dresses will not work for this style of bodywork. It is best for both the practitioner and the recipient to be barefoot. Watches and any jewelry that will interfere with giving or receiving the massage should be removed.

Physical Condition

The person giving the massage should be in good physical condition, as the work is very demanding. An ongoing practice in yoga, chi gong, martial arts, and/or dance is an excellent adjunct. The practitioner ideally should be both flexible and strong. It is also ideal for the recipient to be involved in some kind of physical routine on a regular basis and to stretch before the treatment. The more flexible the recipient is, the more the practitioner can "dance" with his or her body.

It is also important to stretch and strengthen your fingers and wrists before performing the massage. The condition of your hands is crucial. They should be warm, relaxed, and strong. Your fingernails should be short and clean. The hands can be strengthened by doing certain exercises, such as push-ups on the fingertips, working hard wax with your fingers until it is soft, and others. If your hands are generally cold, it is important to find a way to increase the circulation to them through some method such as acupuncture, herbs, and/or chi gong. For a short-term solution, soak your hands in hot water prior to the treatment or take a hot shower or sauna to warm up. Maintain the softness of your hands by applying a good cream when necessary.

The recipient should *not* take a hot bath or sauna for about a half hour prior to the massage because they make the skin too moist to comfortably work on. Also, neither you nor your partner should eat just before the session. For the practitioner, this is because eating diverts some of the energy away from the massage toward the digesting of the food, and you will not feel quite as nimble. For the recipient, Thai massage sometimes uses deep abdominal work, which can be uncomfortable if you have eaten prior to the treatment. It is fine to eat and/or take a bath or sauna any time after the massage.

MEDITATION, PRAYER, AND ASPIRATION

Before giving a massage, it is important to meditate and pray. This will elevate the vibration of both you and the receiver. According to Susan-Jane Beers, "It is believed that energy fields inside and surrounding the body may be changed through prayer, which in turn may affect a person's health."[1]

Remember that giving a massage can be an integral part of your spiritual practice. I have found the following words by His Holiness The Dalai Lama helpful to remember before, during, and after giving a massage:

Here and now, the external and internal facilities are available to us. We have an opportunity to practice the Dharma [the teachings of the Buddha]. We must resolve to generate an altruistic wish to help others. If you already have such a mind you must enhance it. In order to generate such a mind, the most important thing is to pay constant attention. In your daily life, train in regard to the various aspects and objects of the mind of enlightenment . . . concerning yourself more with others than yourself . . . visualize before you the Buddhas and the children of the Buddha as witness. . . . Due to the presence of many external and internal factors, you should be able to cultivate a fresh noble mind and to awaken or nurture the previous predispositions. If you don't have such previous imprints, then it will be a great benefit to establish fresh dispositions.[2]

In numerous Buddhist sutras (discourses attributed to the Buddha and his early followers) there is reference to the Buddha himself studying, practicing, and teaching medicine during his different lives. In this way, the well-intentioned physician's aspiration is considered in accord with dharma practice and can be an integral facet of the altruistic mind of enlightenment. In fact, according to Terry Clifford, doctors practicing Tibetan Buddhist medicine visualize "the medicine mandala for the healing of others. . . . This means one should visualize oneself as the Medicine Buddha and the outer world as the medicine mandala. This is the practice of purifying perception of the world and the self, transforming both into their Buddha-nature. In this case, one is always generating the healing rays of the Medicine Buddha, always generating the best of one's emotional and intellectual capacity as compassion and wisdom in their healing aspects. Realizing the whole of the outer world in its Buddha-nature, it all becomes medicine."[3] Visualizing in this way can be helpful when giving a Thai massage.

THE EFFECTS OF THE TREATMENT

Just as nature always strives to be in perfect harmony, so too does the human body. The process of maintaining relatively stable conditions with respect to multiple organ systems, intra- and extracellular fluids, and tissue functions by internal processes that counteract any departure from the normal is called *homeostasis*. Homeostasis depends on the interconnectedness of numerous systems that receive uncountable inputs. Thai massage supports this natural striving toward balance.

Thomas Hanna, Director of the Novato Institute for Somatic Research and Training, describes this process in regard to the sensory-motor system as follows:

> Any imbalance in the sensory-motor system creates imbalance throughout the entire body. When the muscles in one single limb become spastic or clumsy or too flaccid, this loss of control and efficient coordination within the musculoskeletal system causes an automatic compensation within all the other interconnected bodily parts. The brain brings about these compensations automatically and unconsciously in an attempt to rebalance the entire system.[4]

In other words, homeostasis is occurring.

Thai massage's multifaceted approach to the body and its large repertoire of stretches brings greater symmetry and increased mobility to the musculoskeletal system. Once the musculoskeletal system is more at ease, all the other bodily systems can work more efficiently.

Due to the interconnectedness of all the body systems—skeletal, lymphatic, nervous, digestive, cardiovascular, endocrine, urinary, reproductive, integumentary (the skin, hair, and nails), and respiratory—changes in any one system will affect all the other systems. Furthermore, since structure and function are closely interrelated, if the structure of a body part changes, functions are also affected. A simple movement of the arm at the shoulder illustrates this. In Thai massage, several techniques bring the shoulder joints to the furthest extent of their range of motion in various planes of movement. Most obviously, the muscles are elongated and the ligaments are stretched. However, numerous other effects that are less obvious also occur. Lymph nodes located under the arm are squeezed, aiding the movement of lymphatic fluid on its course to the blood. Nerve function in the shoulder complex is enhanced as surrounding tissues are stretched and the contraction of scar tissue, if any, is diminished. Blood flow to and from the area is stimulated, accelerating the exchange of nutrients and removal of toxins. Synovial fluid, the body's natural lubricant between joint surfaces, is released into the joint cavity to reduce friction between the moving surfaces. Two types of body structures known as *fascia*—one that connects skin to muscle and bone and one that surrounds and separates muscles—are stretched in size. This improves muscle function and circulation. The effect goes beyond the shoulder to also enable increased expansion of the chest wall. Greater volume in the chest cavity allows for fuller expansion of the lungs and, therefore, deeper breathing, which improves the supply of oxygen to all of the body's tissues. And so it goes, on and on and on . . . one system working in harmony with the other to provide the balance necessary for the deeper sense of well-being we all yearn for.

Due to the interrelatedness of structure and function, and of the many systems within the body from the level of microscopic cells to entire organ systems, it is not possible to fully describe the myriad benefits that occur from each technique in Thai massage. Therefore, the benefits that are listed after each technique in Chapter 9 are necessarily incomplete. Only the most obvious physical benefits have been noted. Numerous other muscles, nerves, ligaments, tendons, fascia, lymph nodes, glands, and organs are also affected, as are the mind and spirit. Likewise, the following list is only a partial listing of the many ways that Thai massage can benefit a person. It can:

- Reduce stress

- Reduce pain

- Reduce swelling

- Increase blood circulation

- Increase lymphatic circulation

- Facilitate the removal of toxins

- Increase joint mobility

- Improve flexibility

- Improve body symmetry

- Increase energy flow

- Facilitate contact with unconscious memories

- Facilitate the release of emotional pain

This partial list illustrates many of the ways in which Thai massage can help. For a deeper understanding, one really needs to study in depth how the body is designed and how each system works within it. For this I highly recommend Dr. Krishna Raman's book *A Matter of Health* (East West Books), in which he explains how yoga benefits each system in the body. Other books on yoga, stretching, and massage will give further information on the benefits derived from these practices that can then be applied to Thai massage, as it utilizes all of these forms.

Closure of the Treatment

How you close your session is as important as how you open it. Sometimes it is good to talk after the session or to pray again, and sometimes it is good to be quiet. In any case, it is always important to suggest that the person stay and rest after the treatment. Just as the Corpse Pose (Savasana, a pose of deep conscious relaxation) is so important after a yoga practice because it removes fatigue caused by the asanas and quiets the mind, so is rest important after a massage. While resting, the recipient will more fully reap the benefits of the treatment. It is best if he or she rests in the Savasana posture, which is the posture the Thai massage starts with. Here the person lies flat on his or her back, with eyes closed, arms open with the palms up, and legs straight with the feet dropping toward the sides. Let the person know that you will come back and wake him or her up at an agreed-upon time. Now it is time for you to relax!

THE TRADITIONAL
SEQUENCE: THE
SUPINE POSITION

Whether one believes in a religion or not, and whether one believes
in rebirth or not, there isn't anyone who doesn't appreciate kindness
and compassion.   —HIS HOLINESS THE DALAI LAMA

Welcome now to the actual practice of Thai massage. This chapter
and the chapters that follow have been laid out according to the
traditional sequence used most commonly in northern Thailand. The sequence starts with your partner in the supine position (lying on his or her
back) and then moves on to the side-lying position. From the side-lying position, your partner goes to the prone position (lying on his or her stomach)
and then to the inverted position. The sequence closes with your partner in
the seated position. After that, as mentioned at the end of Chapter 8, your
partner can rest in the supine position in Savasana—the Corpse Pose.

Within each of the sequence's positions, there are many techniques.
These techniques have been given sequentially. Some are basic and some
are optional. The optional techniques are either variations of the basic techniques or additional different techniques. There is a logical flow to the
techniques that you will understand when you do a session. The body is
slowly opened more and more, like a flower opening.

If you use only the basic techniques, the session will take you about one and a half to one and three quarter hours. If you add optional techniques it will, of course, take you longer. Each technique has been illustrated with one or more photographs and its benefits explained. Your creativity and understanding come into play in how you select and combine the different techniques. For example, if someone tells you at the beginning that he or she has a back problem, you should devote a good portion of the massage to the back. Someone else may need more time spent on the legs or shoulders. Your partner's needs and condition, the time available for the session, and your own condition are what determine how the session will unfold. What is given in these chapters is more than enough material from which you can pick and choose techniques to give your partner a very beneficial and healing treatment.

In order to create a session and not just do it by rote, it is important initially to learn all of the basic techniques and then all of the optional techniques in the order that they have been given. After learning and practicing all of the techniques until you feel confident of them, you can pick and choose whichever techniques you would like to use during your session.

Note that the positions described in these chapters are based on giving a massage to a female. Since in Thai massage a female's left side is usually worked on first, the text and photos depict that. Although her right side is usually worked on next, it has not been photographed, as the techniques are the same as they were from the left side. Even though there aren't photos from the right side, do not forget to do the techniques from that side. And remember, if you are working on a man, his right side should be worked on first, followed by work on his left side. Therefore, when you are working on a male, imagine the instructions and photos from the opposite side.

For the sake of visual clarity for this book, the model was asked to move her position sometimes so that the therapist's hands or position could be seen better, although in real life, of course, a recipient would not have to move around except in the transitions from supine to side lying and from side lying to prone and so forth.

May you enjoy the learning process as well as the giving and receiving. Good luck—or *chok dee,* as they say in Thailand.

I. The Supine Position

The Thai massage routine begins in the basic supine position, lying on the back with the arms relaxed by the sides of the body and the palms open. The legs should be straight, with the feet relaxed naturally out to the sides, shoulder-width apart from each other. In yoga, as mentioned in Chapter 8, this is known as Savasana or the Corpse Pose. A small pillow can be placed under the recipient's head if wanted.

People preparing to have a massage usually like to lie down on the futon as if they were going to sleep. They think, "Ah, now I can relax." The supine posture is very inducing to that, and many people actually fall asleep soon after the massage has started. A person can let go when lying on his or her back. Breathing comes easily, and the mat supports all of his or her body weight.

1. Meditate and Pray

Have the recipient lie down on the mat face up. Kneel behind his or her feet facing the head. Bring your hands together in prayer, acknowledging this sacred moment. Traditionally, the recipient also prays at the beginning of the healing session. Pray or meditate in whatever way feels comfortable for each of you. Traditionally, the wai khru is performed at this time. It is chanted by the practitioner as follows (for an English translation, see page 25):

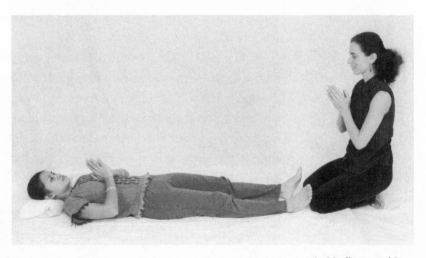

1. Meditate and Pray

Said three times:

Om namoh Shivago silasa ahang karuniko
Sapasatanag osatha tipa-mantang papaso
Suriya-jantang gomalapato paka-sesi wantami
Bantito sumethasso alokha Sumani Homi

Said once:

Piyo-tewa manussanang piyo-poma namuttamo
Piyo-nakha supananang pinisiang nama-mihang
Namo-puttaya navon-navien nasatit-nasatien
Ehi-mama navien-nawe napai-tang-vien
Navien—mahaku ehi-mama piyong—mama
Namo-puttaya

Said three times:

Na-a na-wa lokha payati vina-santi

Two Feet

Techniques 2 through 7 are done on both feet simultaneously. Techniques 2 through 5 mobilize the ankles in all available planes.

2. Palm Press on the Inner Sides of the Feet

This technique relaxes the feet, mobilizes the hip joints, and has an overall relaxing and grounding effect.

Come to a crawling position. Place your palms on the inner sides of the recipient's feet with your thumbs separated from your fingers. Your thumbs should be next to the bones that protrude from the inner ankles. Lean on both feet at the same time as you rock forward and back. Apply your body weight through your arms, which should be straight and at a ninety-degree angle to the inner sides of the recipient's feet. Move your hands down the sides of the feet a little. Your thumbs should now be with your fingers. Lean on the feet again while rocking forward and back. Move your hands still further down the sides of the feet and lean once more. Have most of your weight on the heels of your hands. Bring your hands back to the starting point and repeat. Palm press out the feet three times. The pattern is 1-2-3, 1-2-3, 1-2-3.

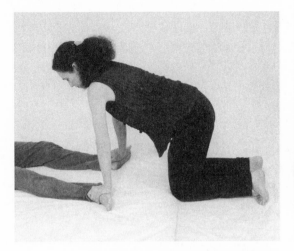

2. Palm Press on the Inner Sides of the Feet

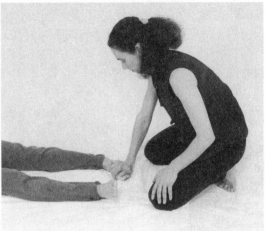

3. Invert the Feet

3. Invert the Feet (Optional)

This technique mobilizes the hip joint.

Drop your hips down so that you are in a kneeling position. Hold one of the recipient's feet and roll it inward. Then roll the other inward. Repeat a few times.

4. Dorsiflex the Feet (Optional)

This technique mobilizes the ankle joint and stretches the Achilles tendon and the calf muscles, specifically the gastrocnemius, soleus, and plantaris muscles.

Hold the balls and toes of both feet and flex the feet backward as far as possible. Relax the pressure and then repeat two more times.

Note: If there is any difference between the lengths of the heels, this may indicate that one leg is shorter than the other or that the pelvis is tilted. In most cases, an apparent difference in leg length is due to the pelvis not being straight. In either case, this may cause problems with the

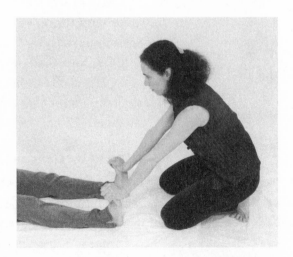

4. Dorsiflex the Feet

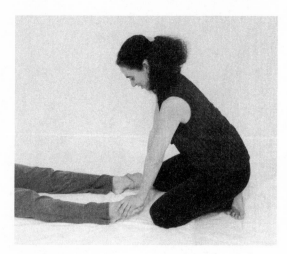

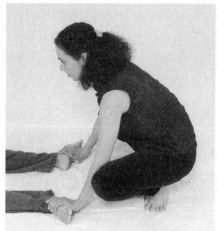

5. Plantarflex the Feet

6. Work Five Lines on the Soles of the Feet

back, spine, shoulders, neck, and/or head as the body tries to compensate for the imbalance. If the problem is due to pelvic misalignment, chiropractic work, massage, and yoga will help. If the problem is actually due to a difference in leg length, orthotics will help.

5. Plantarflex the Feet (Optional)

This technique mobilizes the ankle joint and stretches the muscles in the front compartment of the leg—specifically, the tibialis anterior and peroneus tertius muscles—and stretches the intrinsic components of the foot.

Press down on the top of both feet near the ankles, then at the middle of the feet, and lastly near the toes. Then reverse by pressing at the middle of the feet and then at the ankles. The full pattern is 1-2-3-2-1. Repeat a few times.

6. Work Five Lines on the Soles of the Feet

This technique stimulates Sen Kalathari, relaxes the foot's intrinsic muscles, and stimulates the nerve endings and reflex points on the soles of the feet. It improves general health and revitalizes energy.

Come to a squatting position on the balls of your feet with your knees spread open. (If this position is too hard for you, kneel on the mat.) Place

FIVE LINES ON THE SOLES OF THE FEET

There are five lines on the sole of each foot. Each line starts just above the heel on the midline of the foot and goes out to one of the toes. Line 1 goes to the big toe, line 2 to the second toe, and so forth up to line 5, which goes out to the little toe. These five lines are part of Sen Kalathari. (For a review of the sen, see Chapter 5.)

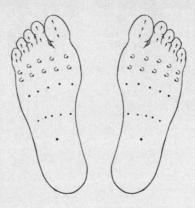

your thumbs just above the heels on the midline of the foot, and with straight arms, lean into the points. Use your thighs to support your elbows. The direction of pressure is up toward the head. Next, thumb press up the insteps of both feet on line 1, going toward the balls of the feet. (*See* Five Lines on the Soles of the Feet, above.) Then thumb circle the balls of the feet on line 1. Finish by squeezing and sliding out the big toes. Repeat the above sequence on lines 2, 3, 4, and 5, consecutively. Remember that each line runs from the starting point, just above the heels, to its corresponding toe.

Note: Not only do the feet have many reflex points and channels running through them, but they also are said to have more than 7,000 nerve endings each. Calcium deposits caused by excess acidity in the bloodstream settle beneath the surface of the skin at the nerve endings of any organ. Due to the abundance of nerve endings in the feet, they are a prime target for these deposits, which can be felt as grainy acid crystals that cause pain when

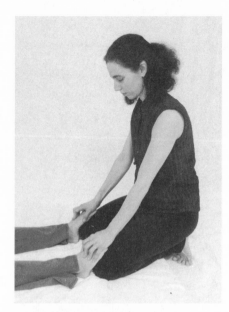

7. Finger Circle on the Tops of the Feet

pressed. These congestions, along with the restricting and sometimes constricting effect of shoes, and the fact that the feet are at the lowest point of circulation, impede normal blood circulation. Toxins therefore tend to stagnate in the feet. Reflexology helps to break down these crystals, which can then be more easily reabsorbed in the blood and removed by the blood circulation.

7. Finger Circle on the Tops of the Feet

This technique relaxes the intrinsic muscles on the tops of the feet. Also, according to Thai belief, it moves wind (energy) down the feet to the toes in preparation for cracking them.

Come to a kneeling position with your knees together. Rest the soles of the recipient's feet on your knees, with the heels turned out a little to stabilize the position. Finger circle on the top of the feet from about the middle of the feet up to just below the toes. Place your thumbs on the inner sides of the feet so that all of your fingers are in contact with the feet as you work. Repeat several times.

One Foot

Techniques 8 through 14 are done first on one foot and then on the other foot. If you are working on a female, do the sequence first on her left foot (her feminine side) and then on her right foot (her masculine side). If you are working on a male, work the right foot first and then the left. This male/female orientation should be continued throughout the treatment.

8. Squeeze the Foot

This technique relaxes the foot and increases its flexibility.

Move to your right. Continue to kneel, but this time have your knees spread open and your hara (center) facing

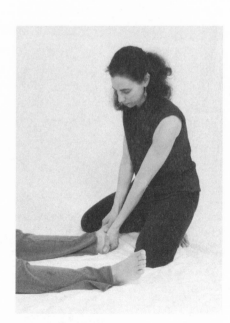

8. Squeeze the Foot

the recipient's left foot. Sandwich the recipient's left foot between your hands, with your right hand behind your left hand. The sandwiching is done between the thenar pad (the fleshy eminence at the base of the thumb) and the fingers. Squeeze the foot from the heel to the toes. Repeat several times.

Note: This is a good way to check the foot's flexibility.

9. Rotate the Foot

This technique mobilizes the ankle joint, stretches the foot extensors, flexors, inverters, and everters.

Swivel your body so that your hara is facing front. Raise your right knee up so that your leg is in a half-squatting position. Your left knee should still be down on the mat. Raise the recipient's foot. Place the heel on the palm of your left hand and lightly clasp the ankle between your left thumb and middle finger. Rest your left forearm on your left thigh. With your right hand, lightly hold the top of the foot from the top. Rotate the foot several times in large clockwise circles. As you do the rotating, move both of your wrists.

Note: This is a good way to check the range of motion of the ankle joint.

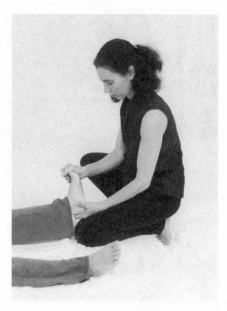

9. Rotate the Foot

10. Twist the Foot

This technique mobilizes the foot and ankle joints and stretches the intrinsic components of the foot.

Continue to hold the recipient's foot with your left hand. With your right hand, hold the inner side of the foot. Twist the foot at the arch, then at the middle of the foot, and lastly at the toes. Do this three times in the following pattern: 1-2-3, 1-2-3, 1-2-3. Then drop your right knee down and raise your left knee up. Exchange the position of your hands so that now your right hand holds the ankle and your left hand holds the outer side of the foot. Twist the foot at the arch, then at the middle of the foot, and lastly at the toes. Do this three times in the following pattern: 1-2-3, 1-2-3, 1-2-3.

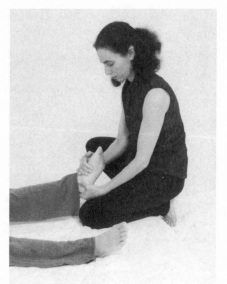

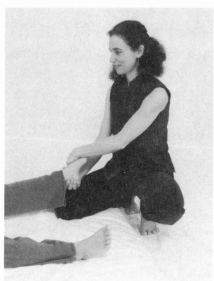

10. Twist the Foot

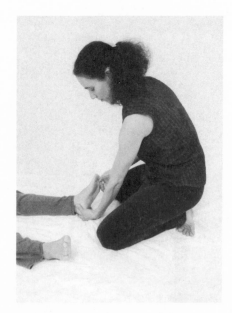

11. Rotate, Pull, and Crack the Toes

11. Rotate, Pull, and Crack the Toes

This technique keeps the toes supple, releases tension in them, and increases space between the joints. Cracking the toes, according to some chiropractors, causes compression of synovial fluid in the joints, which in turn causes the release of nitrogen gas as well as endorphins. According to Thai belief, cracking the toes helps wind (energy) to move into them.

Drop your left knee down. Hold the recipient's foot with your left hand again and bring it down to the mat. Hold the little toe between your right thumb and forefinger. Rotate it a few times. Then give it a quick, dynamic pull. Usually you will hear it crack. If it doesn't crack, don't worry about it. It may mean that you didn't pull the toe strongly and quickly enough or that the finger circling you did on the tops of the feet in Technique 7 wasn't enough. Just go on to the next toe and continue the rotating and pulling on the fourth, third, second, and big toes, consecutively.

Note: The big toe is very hard to crack and often won't crack. Don't worry about this. Also, some people don't like having their toes cracked, so do not do it on them. Also, do not crack the toes if the person has rheumatism in his or her toes.

12. Press Down on the Foot

This technique increases the range of motion of the ankle joint and stretches the muscles of the front compartment of the leg—specifically the peroneus tertius and tibialis anterior muscles—and stretches the intrinsic components of the foot.

Hold the recipient's foot, with your palms on the top of the foot and your fingers below. Keep your arms straight and lean through your arms. Press down first at the ankle, then at the middle of the foot, and lastly at the toes. Repeat three times in the following pattern: 1-2-3, 1-2-3, 1-2-3.

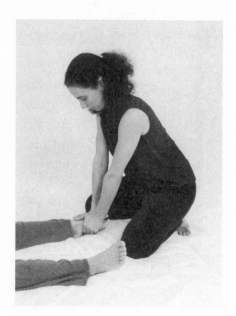

12. Press Down on the Foot

13. "The Wave"

This technique mobilizes the foot, ankle, and hip joints. It also brings in a rhythm establishing trust.

Hold the recipient's foot between both of your hands, with your fingers underneath and your thumbs on the top. With quick flicking movements of your wrists, move the foot up and down. Go from the middle of the foot out to the toes in a wavelike motion. The whole leg should move during this technique. Repeat several times.

14. Massage the Toes Forward (Optional)

This technique stretches the tissues on the bottom of the foot and mobilizes the toes.

Hold the recipient's foot at the toes and massage the toes forward with one hand after the other.

After completing techniques 8 through 14 on one foot, repeat them on the other foot.

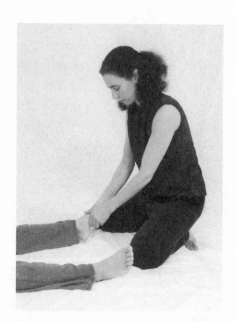

13. The Wave

The Legs

Thai massage really emphasizes work on the legs. In a typical two- or three-hour massage, at least one hour is devoted to the legs. Again this is partly to counteract the effect of gravity. It is also for grounding and because many sen run through the legs. By working on the legs, energy from the sen is released throughout the body. Leg work is also a means of diagnosis and therapy. Problems in the legs indicate problems in other parts of the body, such as the abdomen, back, or shoulders. Ryokyu Endo, a master shiatsu therapist who recommends beginning the treatment by working on the legs, says, "This is because the healer can bring the patient's ki down by performing treatment on the legs which will, to a certain extent, soften any stiffness that may be present in the upper body as well, facilitating treatment there."[1]

There is a joke in Thailand about a foreigner who comes for a massage. He complains of a stiff shoulder. The Thai massage therapist nods knowingly and says, "*Mai phenrai*" (which means "no problem") and begins the massage. The foreigner enjoys it but as time passes wonders when the therapist will ever get to his shoulders. An hour passes, and then two—no sign of shoulder work. Finally, the therapist bows, indicating the massage is over. The foreigner is livid, "What, no shoulder work! I told you I have a stiff shoulder." The therapist smiles, nods again, and disappears. The foreigner walks out disgruntled. Later he notes, "Hm, no shoulder pain," but then reasons, "Maybe I didn't really have shoulder pain after all." Story aside, do keep in mind the profound interconnectedness between the feet, legs, and upper body.

When palming and thumbing the legs, first do the inner side of the leg farthest away from you and then the outer side of the leg closest to you. Then repeat this inner, outer sequence from the other side of the recipient. Remember that for a woman, the left inner leg should be worked on first and vice versa for a man.

15. Palm Press Walk on the Inner Leg

This technique relaxes the foot and leg and stimulates the flow of energy there, which in turn relaxes and stimulates the flow of energy in the upper body. It also prepares the leg for the thumb press walking on the energy lines that follow. It is very grounding.

A. Palm Press Walk on the Foot and Calf

Come to a crawling position with your left knee to the outside of the recipient's right leg and your right knee between the recipient's feet or near the right foot. Have your arms at a ninety-degree angle above the surface that you are working on. Palm press with your right hand at the end of the recipient's left foot by the toes. Then palm press with your left hand inverted on the bottom of the left calf. (Your left hand continues to be inverted while it

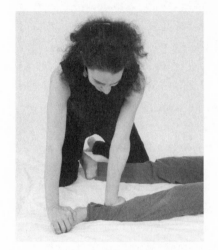

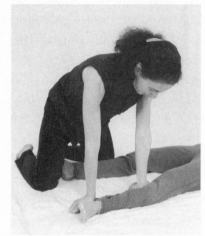

15A. Palm Press Walk on
the Foot and Calf

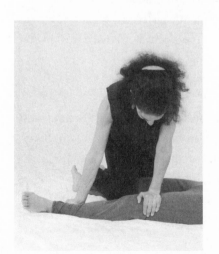

15B. Palm Press Walk up the Calf
and Thigh

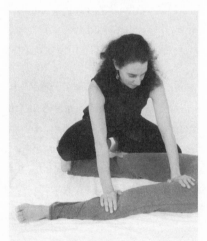

15C. Palm Press Walk
down the Thigh and Calf

is on the calf.) Palm press with your right hand at the middle of the foot, and then palm press with your left hand at the middle of the calf. Invert your right hand and palm press on the heel, and then palm press your left hand at the top of the calf. Then walk your hands down the foot and calf and back up again. The whole pattern is up, down, up.

B. Palm Press Walk up the Calf and Thigh

Move your right knee between the recipient's knees. Move your left hand from the calf to the thigh just above the knee and palm press with your hand straight. Move your right hand from the foot to the calf, keeping your hand inverted, and palm press. (Your right hand continues to be inverted while it travels up the calf.) Continue to palm press walk up the calf and thigh with four more alternate steps, finishing with your left hand at the top of the thigh and your right hand at the top of the calf.

Note: As you palm press walk up the leg the first time, take note of it. This is your "touch diagnosis," so do not press too hard on this round. Then on the second and third rounds, you can apply pressure to those areas where you felt tension. You can increase the pressure by changing the angle of your arms and leaning more. Here it is the thigh, not the calf, that is focused on for applying strong leaning pressure. According to Thai belief, thigh tension, which shows up as hardness or tightness in the area, often indicates lower back or abdominal problems. Strong leaning pressure helps to soften these hardened areas. As you palm press, you are actually working on sen lines that will be thumb pressed later on.

C. Palm Press Walk down the Thigh and Calf

Now lift your right knee and swing it out to the side half kneeling, half squatting on the recipient's right side. Palm press your left hand on the recipient's inner thigh, and your right hand on the inner calf, with both hands straight—not inverted. (Both hands continue to be straight when palming down the leg.) Continue to palm press walk down the thigh and calf. Repeat 15B and C two more times.

D. Palm Press Walk on the Calf and Foot

Come to a crawling position again. Palm press with your left hand at the top of the calf and then with your right hand on the heel of the foot. Continue down with four more alternate steps. This sequence is down, up, down. (See photo 15A.)

THUMB PRESS THROUGH THE JOINT

After palming on the legs, thumbing is performed. In thumbing, the pressure comes through the joint at the middle of the thumb, not through the tip. According to the Thai system of measurement, the length of one finger joint of the index finger is called an *onkkulee*, which is about an inch. When thumb press walking on the lines, the leading thumb slides ahead four onkkulee (about four inches) on the line. The following thumb then "jumps" forward two onkkulee (about two inches) on the line, landing two onkkulee behind the leading thumb. This is continued up and down the lines.

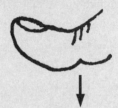

INNER LEG LINES IN THE SUPINE POSITION

The Inner Leg Line 1 (supine) starts just above the inner anklebone. On the lower leg, the line runs on the inner side of the tibia (the shinbone, the main bone of the lower leg). It then crosses the inner side of the knee. On the thigh, the line starts at the inner border of the kneecap and then runs up the thigh just to the inside of the rectus femoris muscle (one of the quadriceps muscles) until it reaches the crease of the groin.

(continued)

The Inner Leg Line 2 (supine) starts next to the inner anklebone. On the lower leg, the line runs up the inner calf, between the gastrocnemius muscle and the tibia. It then crosses the inner side of the knee. On the thigh, the line starts where a small indentation can be felt and runs two onkkulee further inside the leg than Inner Leg Line 1. It stops when the outer side of the leading hand reaches the hip.

The Inner Leg Line 3 (supine) starts on the Achilles tendon just above the heel. On the lower leg, the line runs in the middle of the back of the calf to the back of the knee. On the thigh, the line runs two onkkulee further inside the leg than Inner Leg Line 2.

The easiest way to remember the placement of the inner and outer leg lines in the supine position is to visualize them as parallel streams running from the ankle to the top of the leg. Inner Leg Line 1 runs parallel to Outer Leg Line 1. Inner Leg Line 2 runs parallel to Outer Leg Line 2.

Note: Inner Leg Line 1 is not thumb pressed when doing the leg lines. So the first line that is thumb pressed is actually Inner Leg Line 2.

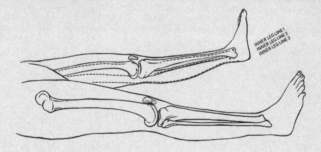

16. Thumb Press Walk on Inner Leg Line 2

This technique stimulates the flow of energy along Inner Leg Line 2.

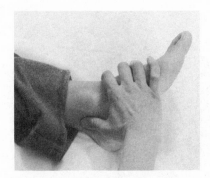

Hold the recipient's ankle with the fingers of your right hand. With your right thumb, press next to the inner anklebone on the starting point of Inner Leg Line 2. Imagine activating energy flow along the whole pathway when you press the starting point. (Visualize this whenever you press any line's starting point.) Then thumb press walk up the calf by the inner side of the tibia on Inner Leg Line 2. Your thumbs should be horizontal and in the line. When you get to the knee, slide your thumbs over the inner side of the knee tracing Inner Leg Line 2. On the thigh, find an indentation and then thumb press walk up the thigh two onkkulee in from the rectus femoris muscle, which is where Inner Leg Line 1 runs. Your thumbs should be at a forty-five-degree angle to the line until the outer side of your leading hand reaches the hip. Thumb press walk down the leg on Inner Leg Line 2 in the same way that you walked up it. Finish by thumb pressing on the starting point of Inner Leg Line 2.

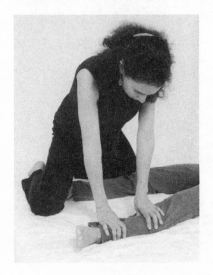

Caution: If the recipient is pregnant, do not press on a point on Inner Leg Line 2 one hand's breadth up from the inner anklebone. This point is known as SP 6 in acupuncture and shiatsu. Activating it can cause uterine contractions.

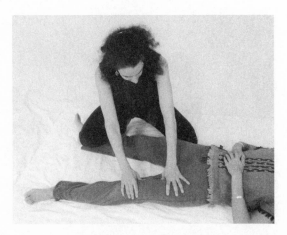

16. Thumb Press Walk on Inner Leg Line 2

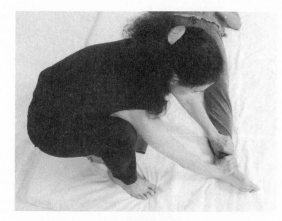

17. Thumb Press Walk on Inner Leg Line 3

This technique stimulates the flow of energy along Inner Leg Line 3.

Hold the recipient's ankle with both of your hands and press with crossed thumbs on the Achilles tendon on the starting point of Inner Leg Line 3. When the Achilles tendon is squeezed with enough pressure, the big toe should move. Thumb press walk up the calf on Inner Leg Line 3 with your thumbs vertically crossing the line. Get strength for your thumb pressure by clasping the other side of the calf with your fingers. When you reach the knee with your right hand, thumb press behind the knee. Then thumb press walk up the thigh on Inner Leg Line 3. Your thumbs should be at a forty-five-degree angle to the line. Thumb press walk down the leg on Inner Leg Line 3 the same way you walked up it. Finish by pressing with crossed thumbs on the starting point of Inner Leg Line 3.

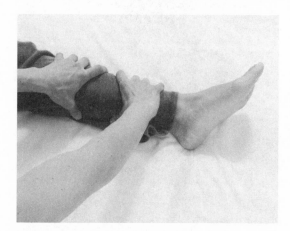

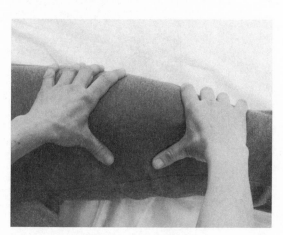

17. Thumb Press Walk on Inner Leg Line 3

18. Palm Circle on the Knee and Thumb Circle on the Inner Anklebone

This technique mobilizes the kneecap and brings energy to the inner anklebone. This is also a way to check the movement of the kneecap.

Palm circle on the left knee with your left hand as you simultaneously thumb circle on the inner anklebone with your right thumb.

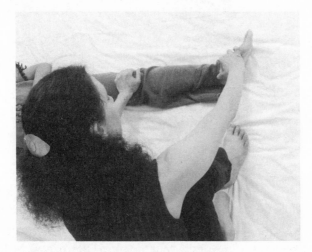

18. Palm Circle on the Knee and Thumb Circle on the Inner Anklebone

After finishing work on the inner side of the left leg, do not go around to the other side of the recipient. Stay where you are and work on the outer side of the right leg.

19. Palm Press on the Outer Side of the Leg

A. Palm Press on the Lower Leg

Half kneel and half squat with your right knee down and your left knee up over the recipient's lower leg. Hold the recipient's right foot with your right hand and roll the leg inward a little to expose the outer side of the lower leg more. Place your left hand inverted just below the knee on the lower leg and palm press down the outside of the lower leg in three steps. Your arm should be at a ninety-degree angle to the top of the calf. Then palm press back up in two steps. Go down and up one more time. The pattern is 1-2-3-2-1-2-3-2-1.

The benefits of the following techniques are the same as those described for step 15.

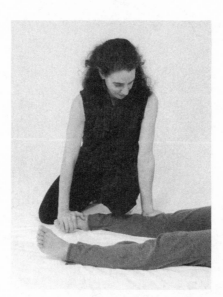

19A. Palm Press on
the Lower Leg

B. Knee Press on the Lower Leg (Optional)

Hold the recipient's leg as you did in step 19A and knee press in small steps with your left knee on the lower leg. Work on the area just below the knee. As you knee press, raise your hips up a little to increase the pressure.

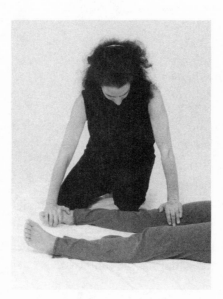

19B. Knee Press
on the Lower Leg

C. Palm Press Walk Up the Leg

Kneel next to the recipient's right leg with your knees wide open. Palm press walk up the calf and thigh. The heel of your left hand should be near the top right side of the thigh. The heel of your right hand should be to the outside of the shinbone. Neither of your hands should be inverted.

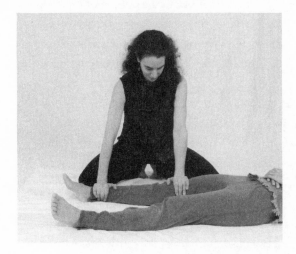

19C. Palm Press
Walk Up the Leg

D. Palm Press Walk Down the Leg

Bring your hands down a little on the outer side of the leg. Palm press walk down the leg. Neither of your hands should be inverted.

Repeat the palming up and down the legs two more times.

E. Palm Press on the Lower Leg

Repeat the procedure in step 19A.

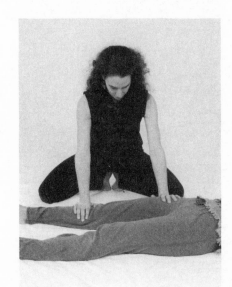

19D. Palm Press
Walk Down the Leg

OUTER LEG LINES IN THE SUPINE POSITION

The Outer Leg Line 1 (supine) starts at the midpoint on the top of the foot, at the transverse malleolus crease between two tendons, the extensor digitorum longus and extensor hallucis longus. On the lower leg, the line runs just to the outside of the tibia on the tibialis anterior muscle. It then crosses the outer side of the knee. On the thigh, the line starts on the outer border of the kneecap and runs up the thigh by the outside border of the rectus femoris muscle to the top of the leg.

The Outer Leg Line 2 (supine) starts below the outer anklebone. On the lower leg, it runs along the lower part of the fibula (the smaller, outer bone in the lower leg). It then crosses the outer side of the knee. On the thigh, the line runs up the outside of the leg on the iliotibial band (a tendon that runs along the outside of the thigh from the knee to the hip). It ends just before the top of the femur (the thighbone).

The Outer Leg Line 3 (supine) on the lower leg is the same as Inner Leg Line 3—it runs in the middle of the back of the calf. It does not run on the thigh in the supine position.

Note: The Outer Leg Line 3 is not thumb pressed when doing the lines in the supine position.

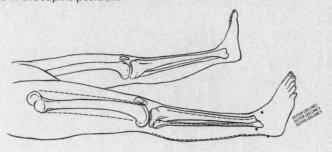

20. Thumb Press on Outer Leg Line 1

This technique stimulates the flow of energy along Outer Leg Line 1.

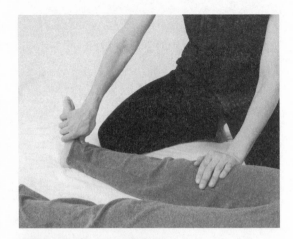

Hold the recipient's right foot with the fingers of your right hand, and with your right thumb, press on the midpoint at the top of the foot between the two tendons, the extensor digitorum longus and extensor hallucis longus, on the starting point of Outer Leg Line 1. Then with your thumbs crossed, press on Outer Leg Line 1 on the lower leg, by the muscle on the outer side of the shinbone. In order to get more strength for your thumb pressure, squeeze the leg between your thumbs and fingers. When you get to the knee area, slide your thumbs over the outer side of the kneecap, tracing Outer Leg Line 1. Thumb press walk up the thigh on the outer border of the rectus femoris muscle, the large central quadriceps muscle, on Outer Leg Line 1 with your thumbs horizontal and in the line. When you get near to the top of the leg, keep the fingers of your left hand stationary and pivot your thumb for hand etiquette to continue walking up Outer Leg Line 1. Thumb press walk down the leg on Outer Leg Line 1 the same way you walked up it. Finish by thumb pressing on the starting point of Outer Leg Line 1.

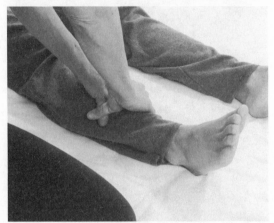

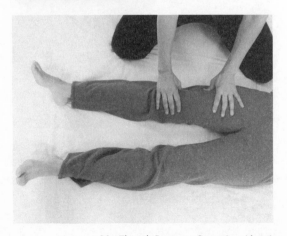

20. Thumb Press on Outer Leg Line 1

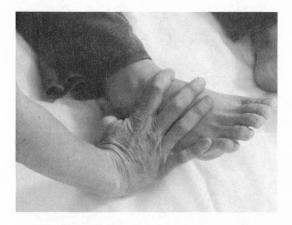

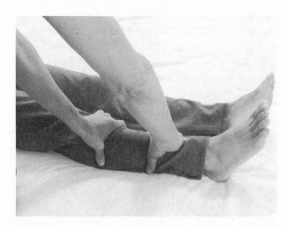

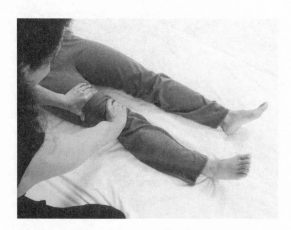

21. Thumb Press on Outer Leg Line 2

21. Thumb Press Walk on Outer Leg Line 2

This technique stimulates the flow of energy along Outer Leg Line 2.

Hold the foot with the fingers of your right hand, and with your right thumb, press just below the outer anklebone on Outer Leg Line 2's starting point. Thumb press walk up on the fibula (the outer, smaller long bone in the lower leg) on Outer Leg Line 2 with your thumbs vertically crossing the line. When you get to the knee area slide over the outer side of the knee with your thumbs tracing Outer Leg Line 2. Thumb press walk up the outside of the thigh on the iliotibial band (a tough band of fibers that runs along the outside of the thigh) on Outer Leg Line 2 with your thumbs vertically crossing the line until just before you reach the greater trochanter (the large prominence on the outside of the hip). When you get near the top of the leg, keep the fingers of your left hand stationary and pivot your thumb for hand etiquette as you continue to walk up Outer Leg Line 2. Thumb press walk down the leg on Outer Leg Line 2 the same way you walked up it. Finish by thumb pressing on the starting point of Outer Leg Line 2.

22. Palm Circle on the Knee and Thumb Circle on the Outer Anklebone

This technique mobilizes the kneecap and brings energy to the outer anklebone.

Palm circle on the right knee with your left hand as you simultaneously thumb circle on the outer anklebone with the thumb of your right hand.

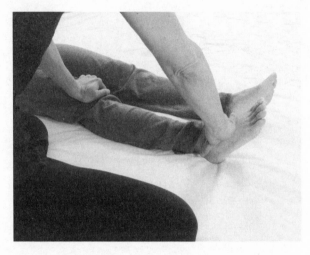

22. Palm Circle on the Knee and Thumb Circle on the Outer Anklebone

Now repeat steps 15 through 22 on the other side—that is, when you have finished working on the inner side of the left leg and the outer side of the right leg, go around to the other side of the recipient and repeat the whole procedure. When you make the transition, do not get up and walk around to the other side of the recipient. Instead, palm press walk on the foot and calf of the right leg as you bring your body around to the other side.

The following leg work is done after the palming and thumbing has been completed on both legs.

23. Sit between the Legs (Optional)

These techniques stop and release the blood, relax the adductors (inner thigh muscles) and quadriceps muscles, and relax the iliotibial band and the tibialis anterior muscle (the muscle on the outer side of the shinbone).

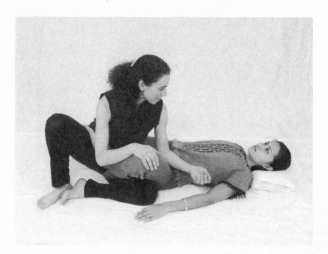

23A. Stop the Blood with the Elbow

A. Stop the Blood with the Elbow

This technique is helpful for knee problems, as it brings a rich supply of blood to this area.

Sit between the recipient's legs, facing the left leg. Have your right knee up. Bend the recipient's left leg and rest it on your left leg, with the foot on your right groin. Place your left elbow on the recipient's left groin over the femoral pulse. Place your right hand on the left knee. Lean on the pulse for sixty pulses. Slowly lighten your pressure. Repeat two more times.

Note: Since the benefits and cautions regarding blood stopping hold true for all blood stopping, they will not be repeated in the descriptions of blood stopping techniques unless there is a benefit that is particular to that technique. See pages 14 through 15 for more information about blood stopping.

B. Press on the Inner Thigh

Place your left forearm on the recipient's left inner thigh near the groin. Lean on the thigh while simultaneously bringing the leg toward you with your right hand. Move your left forearm to the middle of the inner thigh and then lean again while simultaneously pulling the leg toward you. Re-

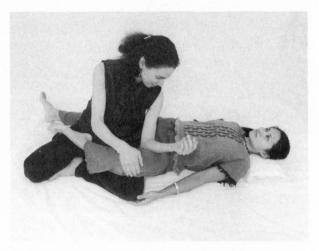

23B. Press on the Inner Thigh

peat with your left forearm just below the recipient's knee on the inner thigh. Then go back toward the groin. Repeat as necessary.

C. Press on the Top of the Thigh

Straighten the recipient's left leg and place the lower leg under your right leg. Place your left forearm on the top of the thigh near the top of the recipient's leg. Lean on the thigh. Repeat with your forearm at the middle of the thigh and then by the knee. Then go back up. Repeat as necessary.

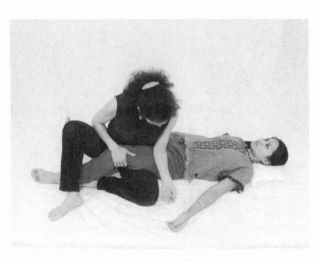

23C. Press on the Top of the Thigh

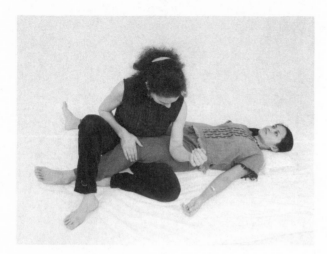

23D. Press the Outer Thigh

D. Press on the Outer Thigh

Place your left forearm on the outer thigh and lean in, moving from the recipient's hip toward the knee and back. Repeat as necessary.

E. Press below the Knee

Move the recipient's left foot out to the side. Move your body down a little. Hold the recipient's foot in place with your right lower leg. Place your left elbow below the knee and your right hand on the lower leg. Lean in on the

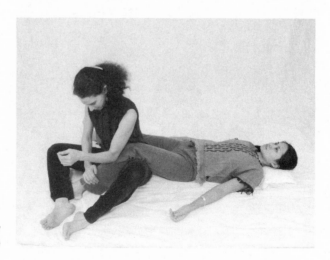

23E. Press below
        the Knee

tibialis anterior muscle (the muscle running along the outer side of the shinbone) with your elbow. Move your elbow to another place below the recipient's knee and lean in. Repeat a few more times.

Repeat the entire step 23 on the other leg.

24. Palm Press Walk Up the Legs and Stop the Blood (Optional)

This technique stops and releases the blood.

Start with the recipient in the original supine position. Kneel between his or her legs and palm press walk up them. Place your hands on both femoral pulses. Lift your knees off the mat and raise your hips up as shown in the photo below. Lean in on the femoral pulses for 180 pulses. Then

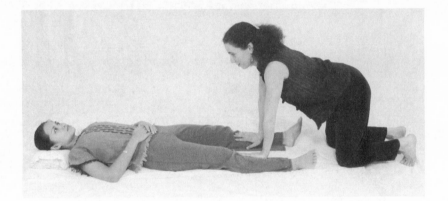

24. Palm Press Walk
up the Legs and Stop
the Blood

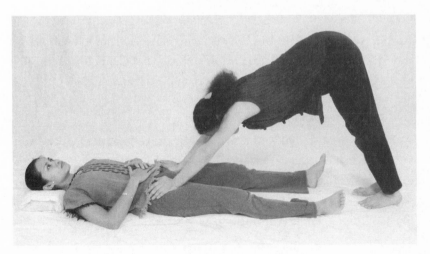

slowly release the pressure from your hands as you bring your knees down to the mat.

25. Leg Bent to the Side

These techniques mobilize the hip and knee joints and stretch the adductor muscles.

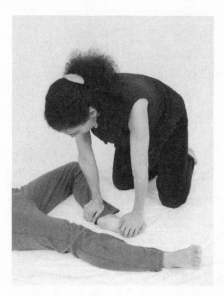

25A. Palm Press Walk on the Foot and Calf

A. Palm Press Walk on the Foot and Calf

Bend the recipient's left leg at the knee. Bring the left foot near the right knee, but keep a little space between them. (If the recipient can't comfortably rest his or her bent leg on the mat, support the leg on your thighs.) Position yourself outside the recipient's lower leg and place your left hand on the left foot, near the toes, and your right hand on the bottom of the calf. Palm press walk up, down, and up the foot and calf.

B. Palm Press Walk on the Calf and Thigh

Position yourself so that your body is facing the recipient's left knee. Move your left hand from the foot to the calf and your right hand from the calf to the thigh. Palm press walk up, down, and up the calf and thigh.

C. Butterfly Hands on the Thigh

Position yourself so that your arms are over the recipient's thigh and your knees are on either side of the recipient's bent leg. Place your hands at the top of the thigh in the butterfly position. (You can modify the butterfly position with your hands spread out a bit from each other.) Press down on the thigh and then lean in at an angle so as to stretch the thigh away from the

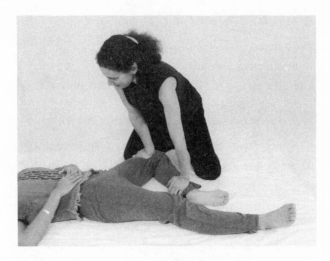

25B. Palm Press Walk on the Calf and Thigh

trunk. Repeat with your hands at the middle of the thigh and then just above the knee. Reverse the butterfly presses, going back up the thigh toward the groin, and then once more down toward the knee. The full pattern is 1-2-3-2-1-2-3.

Note: The pressure should be strongest at the top of the thigh and progressively lighter as you go toward the knee.

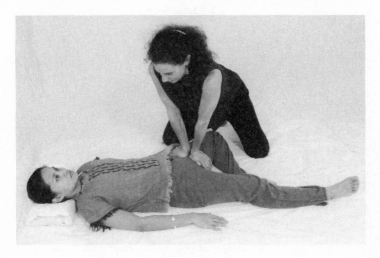

25C. Butterfly Hands on the Thigh

D. Palm Press Walk on the Calf and Foot

Palm press walk down the calf with your right hand and down the foot with your left hand. Go back up the foot and calf and then down one more time. The whole pattern is down, up, down. (See photo 25A.)

26. Foot Press Walk on the Back of the Thigh

This technique mobilizes the hip and knee joints, stretches the adductor (inner thigh) muscles, and compresses the hamstring muscles. It is helpful for people with sciatica and separates the tissues at the back of the leg.

A. Press with the Right Foot

Sit down near the recipient's right lower leg, which should be straight. Bend your left leg and rest it on the recipient's right lower leg. With your left hand, hold the recipient's right ankle. With your right hand hold the left ankle. Begin to push the recipient's left leg forward with your hand and then place your right foot on the back of the left thigh near the knee. With your right foot, continue to push the leg forward until the left thigh is at a right

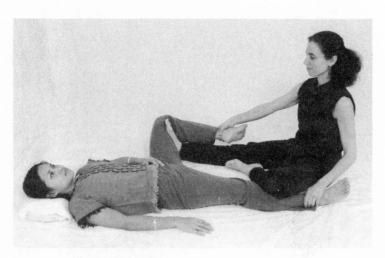

26A. Press with the Right Foot

angle with the recipient's body. Keep your extended leg straight and then pull the recipient's bent leg back toward you against your foot. Put the leg down and draw it a little toward you. Move your right foot in a little on the back of the thigh. Push the recipient's bent leg forward with your foot until your right leg is straight. Then, once again, lean back, pulling the recipient's bent leg against your foot. Repeat with your foot at the middle of the back of the thigh. Make sure that you straighten your leg each time before you pull the leg back against your foot. Then reverse the direction of the foot presses, going back toward the knee. Repeat as necessary.

Note: When sole pressing the first few times here and in step 26E, first feel for areas of tension—don't apply too much pressure. Once you know where the tense areas are, you can apply pressure by pulling the leg more strongly against your foot. Also, make sure to keep your foot vertical; don't let it drop forward.

B. Press with the Outer Side of the Foot (Optional)

With the outer side of your foot, press on the back of the recipient's thigh.

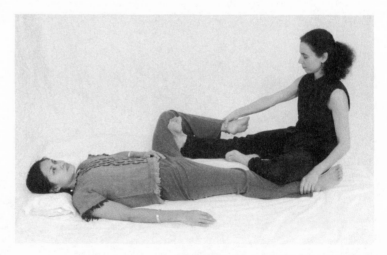

26B. Press with the Outer Side of the Foot

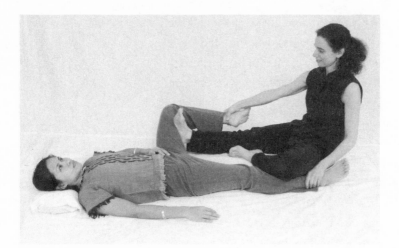

26C. Press with the Heel of the Foot

C. Press with the Heel of the Foot (Optional)

With the heel of your foot, press on the back of the recipient's thigh.

Note: 26B and 26C are methods for increasing the pressure on the back of the thigh.

D. Walk with Both Feet (Optional)

Place both of your feet on the back of the recipient's thigh and walk your feet one after the other.

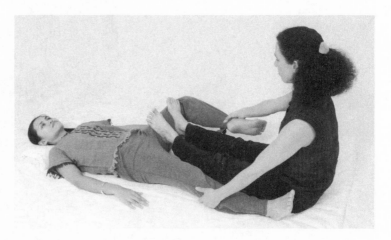

26D. Walk with
        Both Feet

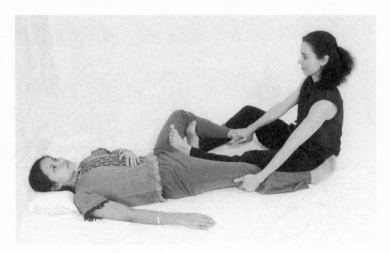

26E. Press with the Left Foot

E. Press with the Left Foot

Interlock the recipient's left lower leg with your right lower leg and, with your right foot, push it as far forward as it will go. Place the sole of your left foot on the back of the recipient's thigh near the groin. Your heel should be about halfway down the thigh and your foot should be vertical; don't let it drop forward. Continue holding the left ankle with your right hand. With your left hand, hold the leg under the right knee. Pull the bent leg toward you against your left foot. Make sure to keep your left leg straight as you pull the thigh against your left foot. Push the bent left leg forward with your right foot and hand. Move your left foot in, going toward the middle of the back of the thigh, and once again, straighten out your left leg as you pull the bent leg against your foot. Repeat with your foot at the middle of the back of the thigh. Repeat the above—pushing the leg forward and then pulling it back against your left foot as you sole press back to the groin. Make sure to straighten out your left leg each time before you pull the recipient's leg back against your foot. Repeat as necessary.

F. Leg Lock, Hook, and Pull

Place both of your feet at the middle of the back of the recipient's thigh. Then place the bent lower leg over your ankles. Lock the recipient's leg in place with your left lower leg and rest your left knee on the extended leg.

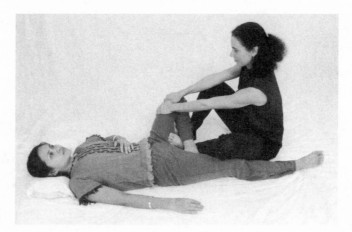

26F. Leg Lock, Hook, and Pull

Move forward so that you are closer to the recipient's bent leg. Place your hands on the recipient's left thigh just above the knee. With your fingertips, hook and pull the leg toward you as you press the back of the thigh with your feet. Repeat with your hands at the middle of the outer thigh and then near the hip. Then do the same thing in reverse. Repeat as necessary.

An alternate way to perform this technique is to hook and pull the leg with one hand after the other.

G. Tapotement (Optional)

With your right hand holding the recipient's knee, hit up and down the thigh with your left hand in a loose fist.

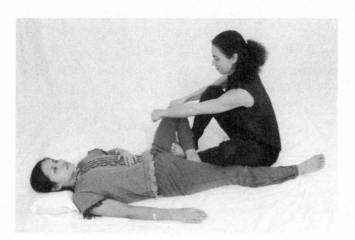

26G. Tapotement

27. Work on the Thigh

These techniques stimulate the flow of energy along Inner and Outer Leg Lines 1 and 2 and mobilize the quadriceps muscles. The pressure on the thigh separates tissues there and stimulates nerve endings.

A. Finger Walk on the Thigh

Move the recipient's bent left leg up so that the knee faces the ceiling and the sole of the foot is flat on the mat under the knee. Stabilize the recipient's bent leg by placing your bent right leg next to it. Rest your left foot on the recipient's left foot near the toes. Place your fingertips on the recipient's thigh, just above the knee, with one of your hands higher up the thigh than the other. The fingertips of one of your hands should be on Outer Leg Line 1 and the fingertips of your other hand should be on Inner Leg Line 1. Walk your hands down the thigh toward the hip, with one of your hands following the other. In other words, if your right hand is in front of your left hand, it should continue to be that way. Do not bring one hand over the other as you walk. Feel for any stiffness on the thigh as you walk. Then walk back toward the knee the same way. Repeat as necessary.

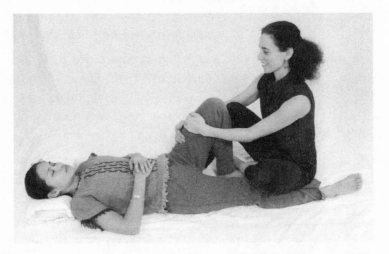

27A. Finger Walk on the Thigh

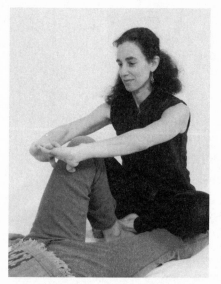

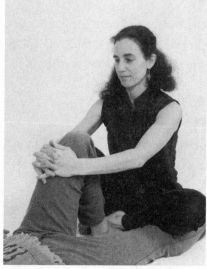

27B. Thumb Squeeze on the Thigh   27C. Hand Squeeze on the Thigh

B. Thumb Squeeze on the Thigh (Optional)

Interlace your fingers. Place your thumbs like pincers on the thigh above the knee on Inner and Outer Leg Line 2 and squeeze. Repeat the thumb squeezes going down toward the hip and then back toward the knee.

C. Hand Squeeze on the Thigh (Optional)

Keeping your fingers interlaced, place the heels of your hands on the recipient's thigh just above the knee on Inner and Outer Leg Line 2. Squeeze the thigh from the knee to the hip and then back again.

28. Pull the Bent Leg Toward You

This technique increases the range of motion of the sacroiliac and hip joints. In the hip joint, the head of the femur (thighbone) is pulled away from the hip socket.

Move the recipient's foot back toward the back of the thigh. Stretch your right leg out. With your fingers interlaced, place your hands above the knee and pull the leg toward you. Repeat with your hands at the middle and then near the top of the thigh. Repeat in the reverse. Repeat as necessary.

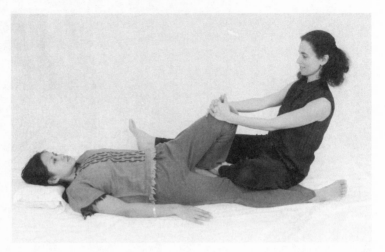

28. Pull the Bent Leg Toward You

29. Thumb Press on the Back of the Thigh

This technique mobilizes the hip joint, relaxes the sciatic nerve, and stretches the gluteus medius (one of the muscles in the buttock).

Move the recipient's left foot out to the side a little so that the knee drops in toward the right leg. Hold the knee down with your left hand. Move your body to the side a little so that you are facing the thigh of the bent leg. With your right thumb, press the back of the thigh from the buttock to the knee and back a few times. Use your right knee as a lever for your right arm to get more strength as you press.

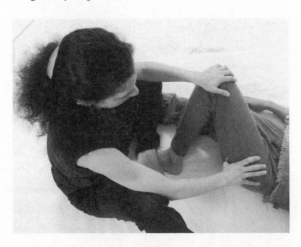

29. Thumb Press on the Back of the Thigh

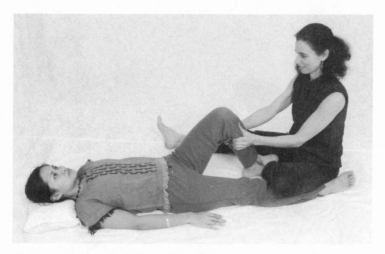

30. Finger Walk on the Middle of the Calf

30. Finger Walk on the Middle of the Calf

This technique relaxes the gastrocnemius and soleus muscles of the calf.

Move the recipient's foot back in toward the extended leg and out toward you so that there is space between the thigh and the calf for your hands. Place your fingertips in the middle of the back of the calf between the gastrocnemius (calf) muscle's two bellies, and your thumbs on the front of the calf. Walk down, up, and again down the middle of the back of the calf as you swing the muscle from side to side. One hand should follow the other.

31. Squeeze the Calf (Optional)

This technique relaxes the calf muscles.

Interlace your fingers. With the heels of your hands, squeeze up and down the calf of the recipient's leg, squeezing it away from the bone.

32. Lift the Heel

This technique mobilizes the ankle joint.

Move the recipient's foot back toward the thigh, so that the heel of the foot is below the knee. Place your right hand on the bent knee and push it forward slightly so that you create a space under the recipient's heel to slide the fingers of your left hand under. Then lift the heel with your fingertips

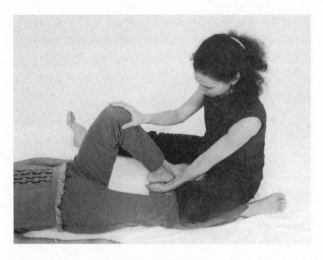

32. Lift the Heel

five times while simultaneously pushing the knee forward a little to help the movement.

33. Bent Leg Up

A. Sole Press on the Back of the Thigh

These techniques mobilize the knee and hip joints, relax the hamstring muscles, stimulate the flow of energy at the back of the thigh, which in turn helps lower back problems, and moves wind into the toes.

Move back a little. Hold the left ankle with your right hand and the foot

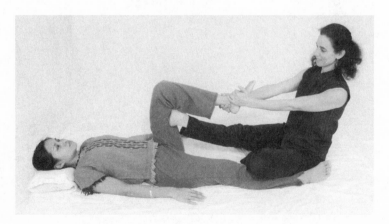

33A. Sole Press on the Back of the Thigh with the Bent Leg Up

with your left hand. Raise the recipient's bent leg up so that the thigh is at a ninety-degree angle to the body. Place your right foot on the back of the thigh behind the knee. Straighten out your right leg. Pull the recipient's leg against your foot while still keeping the bent leg at a ninety-degree angle. With your hands, push the leg forward slightly so that your foot automatically comes a little lower on the thigh. Pull the recipient's leg against your foot again. Repeat in the reverse. Repeat as necessary.

Note: You can also do this with your left foot touching the left ischial tuberosity (the "sit bone").

B. Crack the Toes (Optional)

Hold the ankle with your left hand. With your right hand, pull and crack the toes going from the little toe to the big toe.

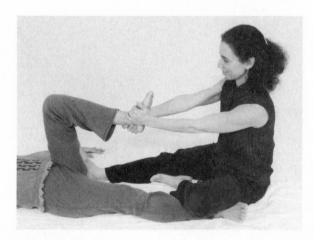

34. Pull the Leg Over Your Foot

This technique mobilizes the hip and knee joints and relaxes the origin of the hamstring muscles.

Place the entire sole of your right foot flat against the back of the thigh of the bent left leg. Hold the recipient's ankle and foot with your hands. Lean back as far as you can pulling the leg over your foot toward you. Sit up as you push the bent leg a little more forward than it was originally. This way,

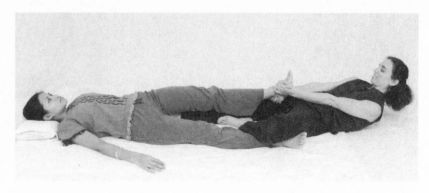

34. Pull the Leg Over
Your Foot

your foot will automatically be lower on the posterior thigh than it was the first time. Once again, pull the bent leg toward you as you lean back as far as you can. Sit up and repeat the procedure. The whole pattern is 1-2-3.

Note: Do not move your foot in this technique. Your foot will automatically end up at a lower place each time due to the increased forward push of the leg.

35. Leg Bent Backward

These techniques mobilize the hip and knee joints, impact the pelvic region, and stretch the quadriceps and psoas muscles. (The psoas muscle runs from the lumbar spine to the thighbone.)

A. Butterfly Press: Standard Version

With your left hand on the knee and your right hand on the ankle, push the left foot back. Then come to a kneeling position. Place your hands in a butterfly or modified butterfly position on the top of the thigh. With your hands in this position, press from the top of the thigh to the knee and back.

Note: If the person you are working on is more than usually stiff or more than usually flexible, use one of the following variations, as appropriate. Do not use these techniques on an individual with any disk or knee problems.

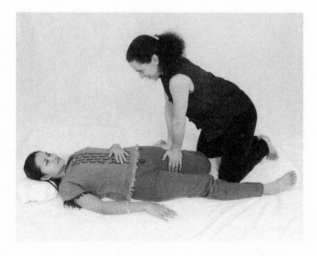

35A. Butterfly Press
with Leg Bent Backward,
Standard Version

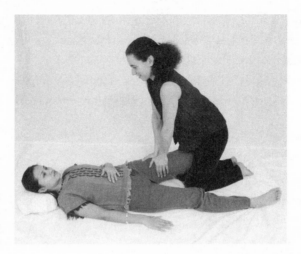

35B. Butterfly Press with
Leg Bent Backward,
Variation for a
Stiff Person

B. Butterfly Press: Variation for a Stiff Person

Rest the leg on both of your thighs or bend your left leg and support the leg on your calf.

C. Variations for a Flexible Person

Variation 1, Knee Press with Hands on Opposite Thigh

Place your knees on the thigh of the recipient's bent leg and place your hands on the thigh of the extended leg.

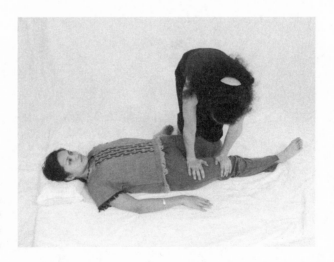

35C. Variation 1 for a
Flexible Person: Knee
Press with Hands on
Opposite Thigh

Variation 2, Knee Press without Hands

With your knees still on the thigh of the recipient's bent leg, raise your hands off of the thigh of the extended leg and raise your chest up so that you are upright.

36. Knee Forward and to the Side

These techniques mobilize the hip and knee joints, impact the pelvis, and stretch the gluteus maximus (a buttock muscle) and adductor (inner thigh) muscles.

A. Hands on the Bent Leg

Place the recipient's left foot above the right side of your groin and come to a half-lunge position with your left knee down and your right knee up. Your left knee should be a little way behind the recipient's

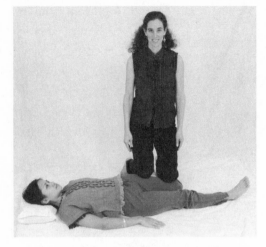

35D. Variation 2 for a Flexible Person: Knee Press without Hands

bent leg and your right foot should be at the side of the recipient's chest. Hold the knee with your right hand and place your left hand on the back of the thigh, near the groin. Make sure to keep your arms straight. Rock your pelvis forward so that the bent leg moves forward, toward the shoulder. The power for this movement should come mainly from your pelvis rather than

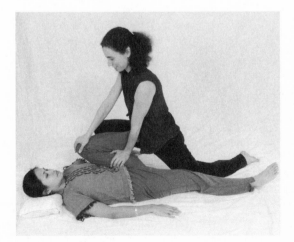
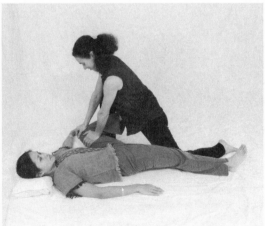

36A. Hands on the Bent Leg with the Knee Forward and to the Side

from your hands, which are there mainly to enhance the movement. Come back. Turn your right foot out to the side forty-five degrees. Bring the recipient's bent leg forty-five degrees to the side. Move your left hand to the middle of the posterior thigh. Rock forward again from your pelvis. Come back. Move your foot further out to the side, which will automatically bring the recipient's bent leg further out to the side, to about a seventy-five-degree angle. Place your left hand near the knee. Rock forward again from your pelvis.

B. Hand on the Extended Leg (Optional)

Begin in the starting position for step 36A, only this time place your left hand on the front of the thigh of the recipient's extended leg and your right hand on the recipient's left knee. Repeat the techniques for step 36A, this time using your left hand to palm press on the extended leg. Repeat with the bent leg out to the side, continuing to palm press on the straight leg.

C. Butterfly Hands on the Thigh (Optional)

Move your left knee to the side and turn your body so that you are facing the recipient. Move your right foot toward the recipient a little. Place your hands in the butterfly position on the recipient's thigh, near the groin. Go from there to the knee and back a few times. To increase your force, stretch your left leg out into a full lunge.

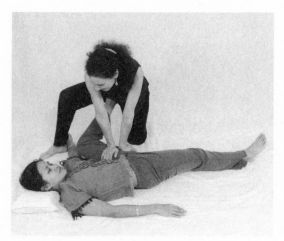
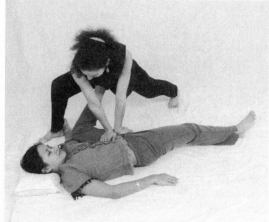

36C. Butterfly Hands on the Thigh

37. Forearm Press (Optional)

This technique mobilizes the hip and knee joints, and relaxes the hamstring and calf muscles.

Come to a half-lunge position at the side of the recipient with your right knee up and your left knee on the mat. Place your right forearm between the recipient's calf and thigh. Hold the left foot with your left hand. Press down on your forearm with the left lower leg. Raise the lower leg slightly and then move your forearm somewhere else and press again. Repeat a few times at different places.

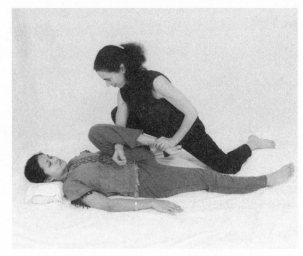

37. Forearm Press

38. Straight Leg out to the Side (Optional)

These techniques mobilize the hip joint, stretch the adductor muscles, stimulate the flow of energy from Inner Leg Lines 2 and 3, and stop the blood.

A. Knee Press on the Inner Thigh

Kneel on your left knee and half lunge with your right leg. Place the recipient's left ankle between your left big and second toes and then slide the leg out to the side with your right foot. Place your left knee on the back of the thigh, near the groin. Hold the front of the thigh with both of your hands. Press in with your knee as you simultaneously pull the thigh against your knee. Repeat the knee press going up and down the back of the thigh.

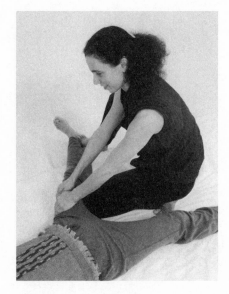

38A. Knee Press on the Inner Thigh with the Straight Leg Out to the Side

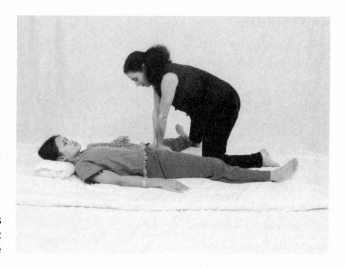

38B. Butterfly Hand Press
with the Straight Leg Out
to the Side

B. Butterfly Hand Press

Raise your hips up and, with your hands in the butterfly position, palm press up and down the thigh of the outstretched leg.

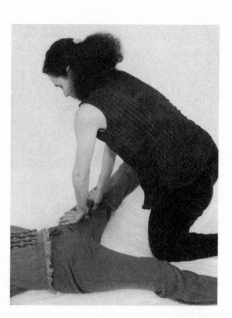

C. Thumb Press Walk on the Lines

Thumb press walk from the groin to the foot on Inner Leg Line 2. This is followed by a double thumb press at the starting point of Inner Leg Line 3 and then thumb press walking from the foot to the groin on Inner Leg Line 3.

38C. Thumb Press
Walk on the Lines
with the Straight
Leg Out to the Side

D. Stop the Blood

Place your left hand on the inguinal crease (the crease at the groin where the leg joins the trunk) over the femoral pulse. Raise your hips up so that your weight can go down through your hand. Rest your right elbow on your thigh so that your right hand is free. Lean on the femoral pulse for sixty seconds. Slowly release the pressure and then repeat two more times.

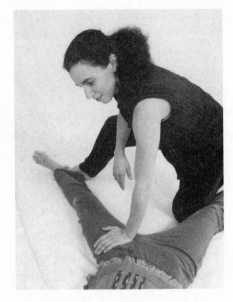

38D. Stop the Blood with the Straight Leg Out to the Side

39. Foot Press with the Straight Leg Out to the Side (Optional)

This technique mobilizes the hip joint, stretches the adductor muscles, and relaxes the quadriceps muscle and iliotibial band.

Come around to the left side and bring the leg toward you. Place your left foot under the left ankle, drawing it in a little closer. Place your right foot on the left hip and press. Then move your right foot to the outer thigh

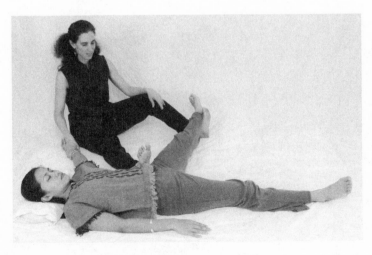

39. Foot Press with the Straight Leg Out to the Side

and press. Repeat the foot presses, going out toward the knee and back a few times. Simultaneously, with your left foot, pull the leg toward you against your right foot.

40. Hamstring Stretch

This technique stretches the hamstring muscles—three muscles in the back of the thigh that work together to flex the knee and extend the thigh—and the piriformis muscle, a small muscle running across the buttock that rotates the hip outward.

A. Standard Version: With the Hand

Come to a half-lunge position with your left knee down and your right knee up. Hold the recipient's left heel with your left hand as you place your right hand inverted on the left ischial tuberosity (the "sit bone"). Stretch the recipient's leg toward the right shoulder. Release the stretch by bringing the foot back toward you. Move your right hand a little way up the back of the thigh and stretch the leg a little more forward than you did the first time. Release the stretch and move your right hand back to the ischial tuberosity. Stretch the leg forward again and then release it. The full pattern of your right hand is 1-2-1.

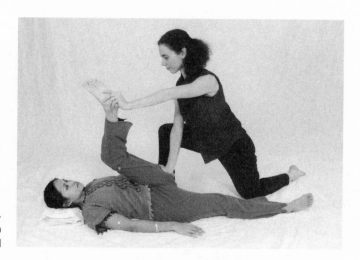

40A. Hamstring Stretch, Standard Version: With the Hand

B. Variation: With the Knee

Repeat the above stretches, but this time place your right knee on the leg instead of your right hand and hold the left heel with both of your hands.

41. Palm Circle on the Knee

This technique relaxes the kneecap and brings energy there.

Come to a half-kneeling and half-squatting position outside the left leg, with your right knee down and your left knee up. Place your right hand under the knee for support as you straighten the leg out. Rest the extended leg on your thigh. Palm circle on the knee with your right hand. Your left hand should rest on the ankle.

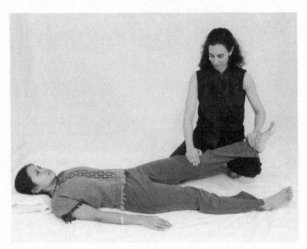

41. Palm Circle on the Knee

42. Diagonal Leg Stretch

This technique flexes the hip joint and stretches the Achilles tendon, the gastrocnemius, soleus, and plantaris (calf) muscles, and the hamstring muscles. It also energizes the lines at the back of the leg.

Come to the outer side of the recipient's left leg. Kneel on your right knee facing the feet. Be on the ball of your right foot. Half lunge with your left leg, with your foot flat on the floor. Hold the left heel with your left fingers. The foot will rest against your forearm. Place your right hand on the lower leg, near the ankle, with your right forearm resting lightly against the leg. Raise the leg up. Lean back. Next drop your right foot down so that the top of your foot is flat on the mat so that you can sit lower. Slide your right hand down to the middle of the lower leg and lean back a little further. Then slide your right hand down to just above the knee. Lean back still further.

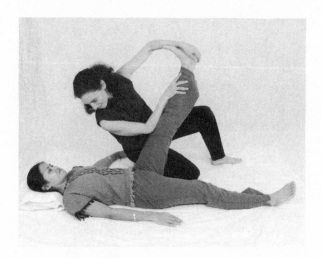

42. Diagonal Leg Stretch

43. Straight Leg Stretch

These techniques flex the hip joint, stretch the hamstring and gastrocnemius muscles, and energize the lines at the back of the leg.

Note: If the person you are working on is very stiff or very flexible, use one of the variations below, as appropriate.

A. Standard Version

Kneel by the recipient's legs facing the head. Raise the left leg straight up. Lightly place your left knee on the thigh of the right leg to stabilize it. Hold the left heel with your right hand and place your left hand just above the knee. Stretch the leg forward with your right hand. Release the stretch by bringing the leg back a little. Move your left hand to the middle of the thigh. Stretch the leg a little further forward with your right hand. Release the stretch by bringing the leg back again a little. Move your left hand further down near the top of the thigh. Once again stretch the leg forward with your right hand. This time, as you stretch the leg, raise your hips up so that you can stretch the leg further forward.

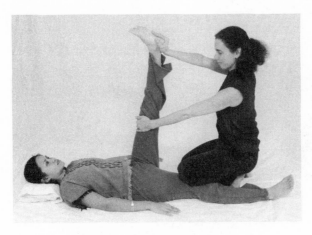

43A. Straight Leg Stretch

B. Variation for a Stiff Person

Kneel on your left knee and half lunge with your right leg. Place the recipient's left ankle on your right shoulder. Place your hands on the thigh. Slowly raise your body up, stretching the leg. If the person is flexible enough to permit it, raise your body up almost to a standing position and place your left foot on the right thigh. Lean forward to increase the stretch.

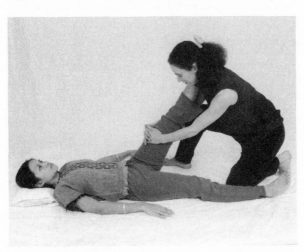

43B. Straight Leg Stretch, Variation for a Stiff Person

C. Variation for a Flexible Person

Stand up and place your left foot on the recipient's right foot to prevent that leg from coming off of the mat. Hold the left heel with your left hand and

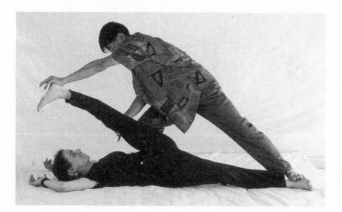

43C. Straight Leg Stretch, Variation for a Flexible Person

place your right hand just above the knee. Stretch the leg forward as much as you can.

Once you have completed techniques 25 through 43 on one side of the recipient's body, go back and repeat them on the other side.

44. Cobbler's Pose (Optional)

These techniques stretch the adductor muscles and open the hip joints.

A. With Hands on the Knees

Bend both of the recipient's legs at the knees and place the feet together. Let the knees drop down toward the mat. Kneel with your knees on either side

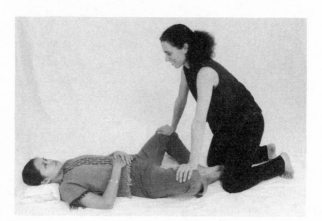

44A. Cobbler's Pose with
Hands on the Knees

of the feet. Place your hands on the recipient's knees and then lean in so that your weight further opens the knees to the sides.

B. Knee Press on the Thighs

Place your knees on the recipient's inner thighs, near the groin area. With your hands, hold the outsides of the thighs. Knee press walk from the groin area out toward the knees and back.

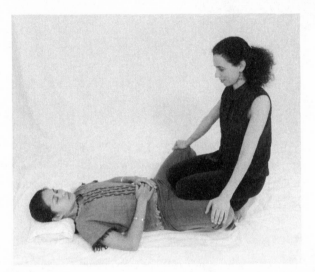

44B. Cobbler's Pose with Knee Press on the Thighs

C. Pull Thighs against Your Knees

Knee press walk with both of your knees simultaneously from the groin out to the knees and back. As you knee press, pull the thighs up against your knees.

45. Spinal Twist from the Right Side (Optional)

This technique improves spinal and hip mobility and stretches the latissimus dorsi (a broad lower back muscle) and piriformis muscle of the buttock.

Straighten your partner's legs. Then

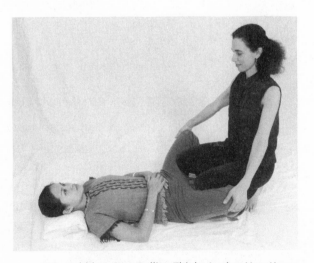

44C. Cobbler's Pose Pulling Thighs Against Your Knees

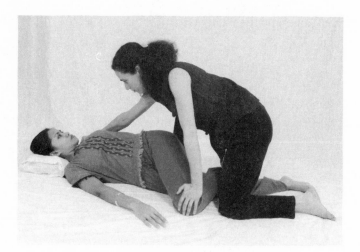

45. Spinal Twist from the Right Side

come to the right side of the recipient. Half lunge over his or her body. Bend the left leg at the knee. Hold it with your left hand. Bring it across the extended right leg and down to the mat on the opposite side while holding the left shoulder down with your right hand.

46. Spinal Twist from the Left Side (Optional)

This technique improves spinal and hip mobility and stretches the latissimus dorsi (lower back) and piriformis (buttock) muscles.

Kneel at the left side of the recipient. Bend the left leg. Place your right hand on the left shoulder and your left hand on the knee. Push the knee away from you so that the knee goes down to the mat on the right side.

47. Spinal Twist with Leg Lock (Optional)

This technique improves spinal and shoulder mobility; opens the hip joint; mobilizes the shoulder blade; stretches the adductor (inner thigh), latissimus dorsi (lower back), and rhomboid (muscle between shoulder blade and spine) and trapezius (upper back muscles); and stretches the fascia (fibrous connective tissue) of the back.

Sit down on the left side of the recipient. Bend the right leg and interlock the lower leg with your left lower leg. Hold the right arm with both of your hands and pull it toward you. After you have pulled the arm as far as

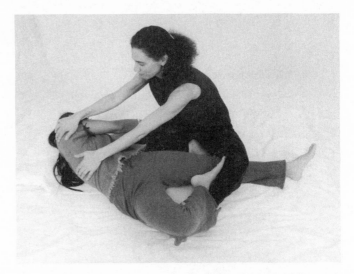

47. Spinal Twist with Leg Lock

you can, hold below the shoulder blade with both of your hands and pull toward you. Then move your hands lower down the back and pull again.

Once you have completed techniques 45, 46, and/or 47 on one side of the recipient's body, repeat the same ones on the other side.

The Abdomen

Thai people believe that the abdomen is the center of the body—that it is a window that reveals intimately what is happening inside. According to author Maxine Shapiro, it "is the home of the breath, the spirit (Qi and Ki) . . . and the energy pump for the whole body."[2] Since this area contains so many vital organs, great care should be taken when working here. Begin with light contact and gradually increase the pressure. If the abdominal tension is too much, have the recipient bend his or her legs. This will soften the abdomen. Make sure to work slowly and sensitively.

You should not do any abdominal work on a person who has just eaten. It also should not be done on pregnant women or anyone with high blood pressure or gastric or duodenal ulcers due to the possibility of hemorrhage.

EIGHT SECTIONS OF THE ABDOMEN

The abdomen can be divided into eight sections. They are normally worked on clockwise, but if a person has diarrhea, they can be worked on counterclockwise. All of the abdominal techniques improve blood supply to the abdominal organs.

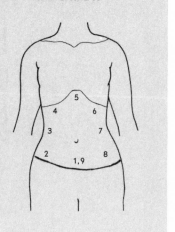

48. Palm Press on the Abdomen (Optional)

This technique relaxes the abdomen and helps peristalsis (the natural rhythmic movement of the intestines).

Kneel by the right side of the recipient. Imagine the recipient's abdomen divided into eight sections, like a pie. (See illustration above.) Place your right hand on the abdomen above the pubic bone with the heel of your hand just above the pubic bone and your fingers pointed toward the navel. Place your left hand across your right hand. As the recipient exhales, sink the heel of your right hand in, pressing toward the navel. As he or she inhales, slightly lighten your pressure. Repeat this for one or two more breaths. Then move your hands clockwise to the next section and repeat. Continue like this, repositioning your hands through all eight sections of the abdomen. At some sections it may feel uncomfortable to use your left hand. In that case only use your right hand. End where you began by repeating the pressure above the pubic bone.

Note: You may find it more comfortable to do the left side of the recipient's abdomen from the left side, which is fine.

49. Push and Pull the Abdomen (Optional)

This technique relaxes the abdomen and helps peristalsis in the intestines.

Kneel facing the recipient's abdomen. Place both of your hands at the

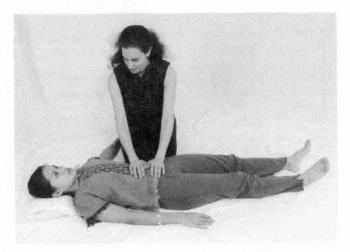

49. Push and Pull the Abdomen

side of the abdomen. With the heels of your hands, push the abdomen away from you. Then, with your fingertips, pull the abdomen toward you. Repeat this back-and-forth motion several times.

50. Abdominal Work while Sitting on the Knees (Optional)

This technique relaxes the abdomen and helps peristalsis in the intestines.

Bend the recipient's legs at the knees and place the feet close to the buttocks. Step over his or her body. Lean over. Place your hands under the re-

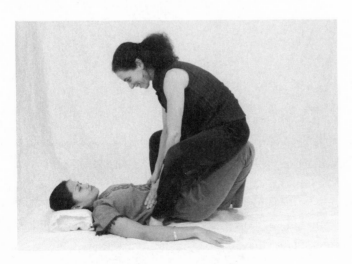

50. Abdominal Work while Sitting on the Knees

cipient's waist and lift it up enough so that you can slide your ankles under the waist. Sit down on the knees. Finger and/or thumb press slowly into the abdomen.

51. Toes in the Abdomen (Optional)

This technique compresses the organs and helps peristalsis in the intestines.

Have the recipient sit up. Hold the recipient's hands with your hands and place your toes in the abdomen. Pull the recipient toward you over your toes. Release a little and then move your toes to another place on the abdomen. Pull the recipient toward you again. Repeat with your toes in other places in the abdomen.

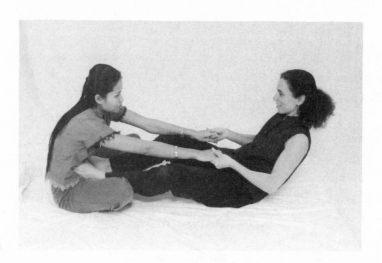

51. Toes in the Abdomen

The Chest

52. Lift the Back (Optional)

This technique mobilizes the spine, relaxes the lower back muscles, and stimulates the flow of energy along the Back Line.

Come to a half-lunge position over the recipient's body, with your right foot by the left hip. Place your fingertips at waist level on either side of the spine. Lift up the back. Move your fingertips higher up the back and repeat. Continue at different places on the lumbar (lower) back.

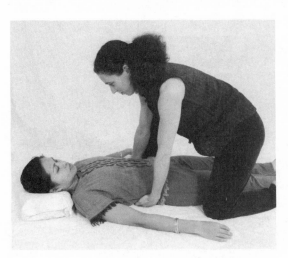 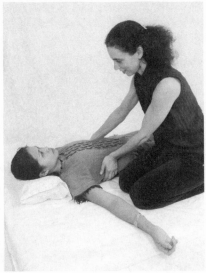

52. Lift the Back   53. Palm Circle on the Sides of the Chest

53. Palm Circle on the Sides of the Torso (Optional)

This technique relaxes the sides of the torso and the muscles there—specifically the serratus anterior and external oblique muscles—and facilitates improved circulation to the area.

Kneel by the right side of the recipient. Palm circle up and down the sides of the torso. Repeat a few times.

54. Hands on the Sternum (Optional)

This technique relaxes the sternum (breastbone).

Join your two palms together and place your hands on the recipient's sternum. Move up the sternum in this way.

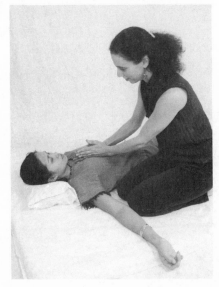

54. Hands on the Sternum

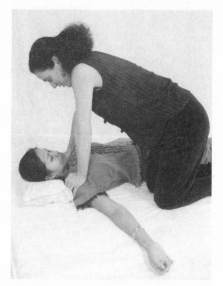

55. Palm Press on the Shoulders

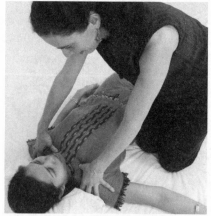

56. Thumb Press Below the Collarbones

55. Palm Press on the Shoulders (Optional)

This technique relaxes the shoulders and the chest muscles, specifically the pectoralis major muscles.

Lift your hips up. Place your hands on the recipient's shoulders and then palm press one shoulder after another.

56. Thumb Press Below the Collarbones (Optional)

This technique relaxes the top of the chest and the muscles there, specifically the pectoralis major muscles.

Thumb press below the collarbones, moving from the center out and back a few times.

57. Raise the Shoulders with Your Hands (Optional)

This technique relaxes the shoulders and the muscles there, specifically the upper trapezius muscles.

Come to a half-lunge position with your right

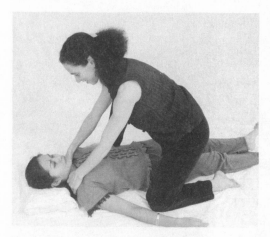

57. Raise the Shoulders with Your Hands

foot over the recipient's body beside the left hip. Place your fingers under the shoulders and pull them up toward you. Repeat a few times.

The Arm and Hand

58. Sole Press on the Front of the Arm (Optional)

This technique relaxes the front of the arm.

Stand up and sole press on the front of the recipient's arm with the ball of your right foot.

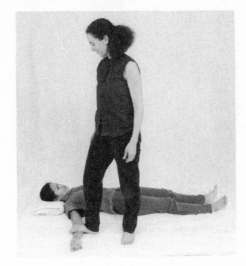

58. Sole Press on the Front of the Arm

59. Palm Press Walk on the Front of the Arm (Optional)

This technique relaxes the front of the arm.

Place the recipient's left arm out to the side with the palm open. Come to a kneeling position and place your left hand on the shoulder and your right hand on the forearm below the elbow. Palm press walk your hands out and back—your left hand will go from the shoulder out to the elbow and back; your right hand will go from the elbow out to the wrist and back.

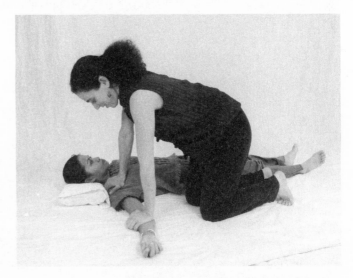

59. Palm Press Walk on the Front of the Arm

THE FRONT ARM LINE IN THE SUPINE POSITION

The Front Arm Line starts at the middle of the inner wrist. On the forearm, it runs on the inner side between the radius and the ulna (the two forearm bones). On the upper arm, it runs along the inside of the biceps muscle up to the armpit.

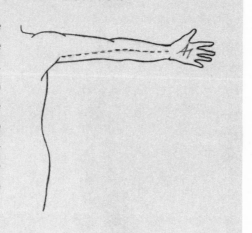

60. Thumb Press Walk on the Front Arm Line (Optional)

This technique stimulates the flow of energy along the Front Arm Line.

Thumb press walk with one thumb after the other from the wrist to the armpit on the Front Arm Line and then return.

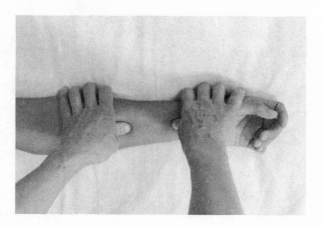

60. Thumb Press Walk on the Front Arm Line

THE BACK ARM LINE

The Back Arm Line starts at the middle of the back of the wrist. On the forearm, it runs on the back side between the radius and the ulna (the two forearm bones). On the upper arm, it runs along the outside of the humerus (upper arm bone) to the top of the arm.

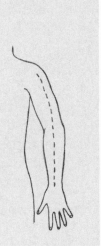

61. Palm Press Walk on the Back of the Arm (Optional)

This technique relaxes the back of the arm.

Turn the recipient's arm over and bring it to the side of the body, with the palm down on the mat. Kneel with your knees open, facing the arm. Palm press walk from the shoulder to the elbow with your right hand as you alternately palm press walk from the elbow to the wrist with your left hand. Then palm press walk back.

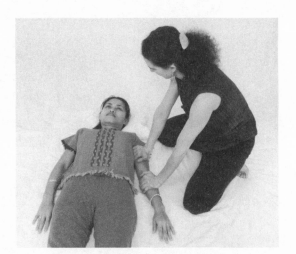

61. Palm Press Walk on the Back of the Arm

62. Thumb Press Walk on the Back Arm Line (Optional)

This technique stimulates the flow of energy along the Back Arm Line.

Thumb press walk with one thumb after the other from the wrist to the top of the arm on the Back Arm Line and then return.

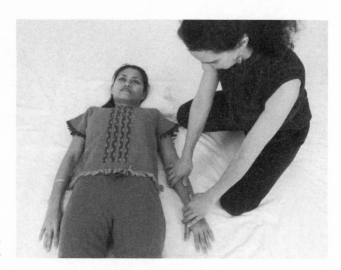

62. Thumb Press Walk on
    the Back Arm Line

63. Thumb Press Five Lines on the Hand (Optional)

This technique stimulates Sen Kalathari, relaxes the intrinsic muscles and nerves on the palms, and affects the reflex points on the palms that affect the corresponding areas of the body.

Turn the recipient's palm so that it faces up. Interlace your fingers from above with the recipient's fingers as follows:

FIVE LINES ON THE PALM OF THE HAND

There are five lines on the palm of each hand. Each line goes from the heel of the hand out to a finger, like a fan. These five lines are part of Sen Kalathari.

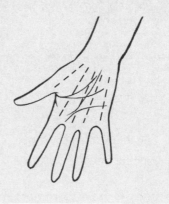

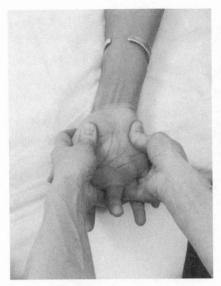

63. Thumb Press Five Lines on the Hand

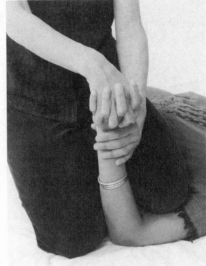

64. Rotate the Hand

- Slide your right pinkie between the recipient's middle and index finger.

- Slide your right ring and middle finger between the index finger and thumb.

- Slide your left pinkie between the recipient's middle and ring finger.

- Slide your left ring finger between the ring finger and pinkie. This leaves the middle finger free.

Thumb press with both of your thumbs simultaneously from the heel of the hand to the base of the thumb and pinkie. Then thumb press to the index and ring fingers. Lastly, thumb press with both of your thumbs to the middle finger. Repeat the thumb pressing down the palm a few more times.

64. Rotate the Hand (Optional)

This technique mobilizes the wrist joint and stimulates the hand flexor and extensor muscles.

Come to a kneeling position, with your right knee on the mat by the elbow and your left knee lightly pressing on the left forearm near the elbow.

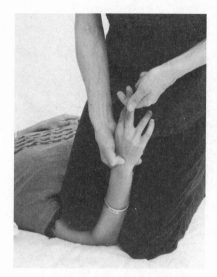

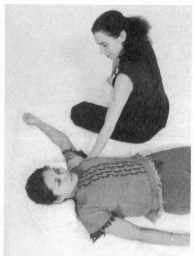

65. Rotate, Pull, and Crack the Fingers   66. Stop the Blood at the Armpit

Interlace the fingers of your right hand with the fingers of the recipient's right hand. Hold the wrist with your left hand. Rotate the hand.

65. Rotate, Pull, and Crack the Fingers (Optional)

Rotating the fingers keeps the fingers supple. For notes on the cracking, see technique 11 on page 82.

With the index and middle finger of your right hand, clasp the recipient's middle finger near the end and rotate it. Then move your fingers in and clasp at the base of the finger. Give a quick pull as you try to crack the finger. Repeat with the pinkie, ring finger, index finger, and then the thumb.

66. Stop the Blood at the Armpit (Optional)

This technique stops and releases the blood.

Sit down by the left side of the recipient, facing the head. Place the arm out to the side. Place your left hand on the armpit and lean in on the brachial artery to stop the blood. Lean for sixty seconds. Release and then repeat two more times.

Note: When you are stopping the blood at the right armpit, do not sit facing the recipient's head—face away from it. Use your left hand again to stop the blood at the brachial artery.

67. Palm Press (Optional)

These techniques open the chest, stretch the latissimus dorsi (upper back) and pectoralis (chest) muscles, and clear the lymph nodes in the armpit.

A. In the Armpit

Kneel on the left side of the recipient with your knees spread open. Bring the left arm back overhead and rest it on the mat or on your knee. Palm press with the heel of your inverted hand in the armpit.

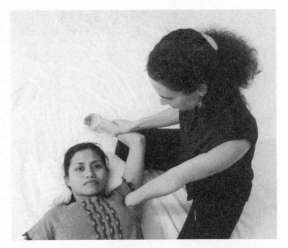

67A. Palm Press in the Armpit

B. Below the Armpit

Palm press with the heel of your hand below the armpit.

68. Thumb Press (Optional)

This technique stretches the latissimus dorsi muscle.

A. In the Armpit

With your thumbs crossed, press in the armpit.

B. Below the Armpit

With your thumbs *not* crossed, press along the side of the rib cage.

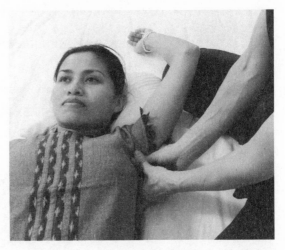

68A. Thumb Press in the Armpit

69. Move the Arm Back and Forth while Working Sensitive Points (Optional)

This technique mobilizes the shoulder joint.

Hold the recipient's forearm with your right hand. Slide your left hand under the shoulder blade, and with your middle finger, find a sensitive point (there are several sensitive points). Press up on that point as you move the arm back toward the head. Then release the pressure as you bring

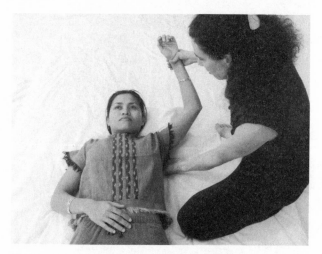

69. Move the Arm Back and Forth While Working
Sensitive Points

the arm back down. Repeat a couple of times and then find another sensitive point and repeat.

70. Pull the Shoulder Blade Out (Optional)

These techniques place traction on the shoulder blade. They also stretch
and relax the rhomboids, levator scapula, erector spinae, latissimus dorsi,
and trapezius muscles.

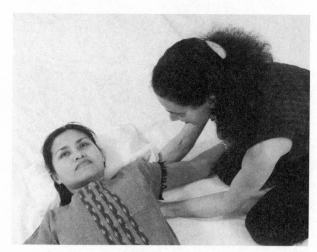

70A. Pull the Shoulder Blade Out with Both Hands

A. With Both Hands

Place the recipient's arm out on the mat at
a ninety-degree angle to the body. Slide
both of your hands under the shoulder
blade and then hook the inner side of the
shoulder blade, drawing it toward you.
Pull and release the shoulder blade a few
times.

B. Work the Erector Spinae Muscles

With the fingertips of your right hand,
continue to pull the shoulder blade toward

you. With the fingertips of your left hand, push up between the spine and the erector spinae muscles (the muscles that run along the side of the spine) on the left side of the back. Then pluck over the erector spinae muscles up and down the back.

71. Triceps Stretch (Optional)

This technique mobilizes the shoulder, elbow, and wrist joints, and stretches the triceps and the wrist flexor muscles.

Bend the recipient's left arm at the elbow. Place the hand palm down on the mat, with the fingers facing the shoulder. With your right hand, hold the elbow, and place your left hand on the hip. Then press the elbow and hip in opposite directions.

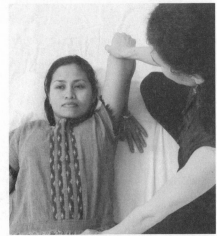

71. Triceps Stretch

72. Arm Rotation (Optional)

This technique mobilizes the shoulder joint and stimulates the muscles there, specifically the rhomboids, pectoralis muscles, and rotator cuff muscles.

With your left hand, hold the recipient's hand, and with your right hand, hold the elbow. Rotate the arm in large circles, pivoting at the shoulder by bringing the elbow up along the mat and then near the face and finally across the left of the torso. Repeat several times.

73. Shake the Arm (Optional)

This technique loosens the shoulder and stimulates blood flow.

Kneel at the recipient's side. Hold the hand and then shake the arm.

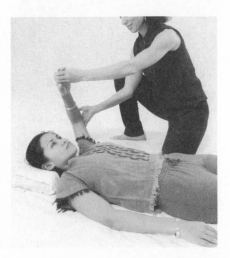

72. Arm Rotation

After completing techniques 58 through 73 on one side of the recipient's body, repeat them on the other side.

The Neck

74. Finger Press the Side of the Neck and Shoulder (Optional)

This technique relaxes the neck and relaxes the muscles there, specifically the scalene, sternocleidomastoid, and trapezius muscles. It also mobilizes the cervical spine (the spine at the neck).

Sit down at the head of the recipient. Turn the head to the left side and rest it on your left hand. With the fingers of your right hand, press the right side of the neck and shoulder.

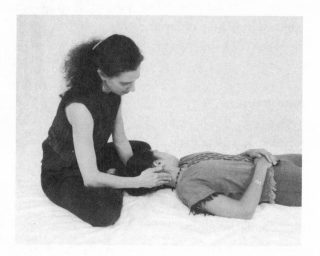

74. Finger Press the Side of the Neck and Shoulder

75. Head Turned, Thumb Press below the Collarbone (Optional)

This technique improves the mobility of the neck and relaxes the pectoralis muscles of the upper chest.

Keep the recipient's head turned to the left side and hold it in place with the fingers of your left hand. With your right thumb, press in different places below the collarbone.

After doing techniques 74 and 75 on one side of the recipient's body, repeat them on the other side.

76. Thumb Press below the Collarbones (Optional)

This technique relaxes the chest and the pectoralis major and minor muscles.

Press with both of your thumbs below the collarbones.

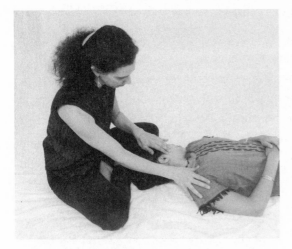

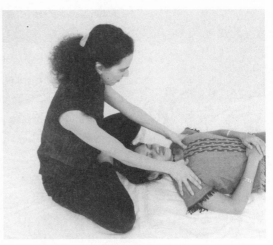

75. Head Turned, Thumb Press below the Collarbone

76. Thumb Press below the Collarbones

The Head

The head, including the face, is usually done in the sitting position in the northern style of Thai massage. Most of the photos for the head massage have therefore been taken in the sitting position. However, many people do the head in the supine position, so I have included the written instructions for massaging the head here as well. I have found that the head massage is more relaxing in the supine position.

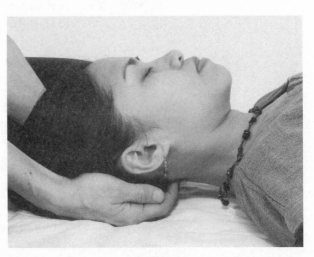

77. Finger Circle on the Occipital Ridge (Optional)

The occipital ridge is the area at the base of the skull. This technique relaxes the upper trapezius muscles, which attach at the base of the skull. It is helpful for headaches.

With your fingertips, circle on the occipital region. Primarily use your middle fingers for this work.

77. Finger Circle on the Occipital Ridge

78. Massage the Scalp (Optional)

This technique stimulates the scalp and hair roots and relieves tension in the head. It can help certain headaches.

With your fingertips, massage the recipient's scalp. To reach the back of the scalp, hold the recipient's head with one of your hands and turn the head to the side. Massage the exposed area with your other hand. Then turn the head to the other side and repeat.

79. Massage the Forehead (Optional)

This technique relaxes the forehead and can help certain headaches.

Finger circle on the forehead from the midline out. Repeat several times, each time at a different place on the forehead. (See photo 191 on page 237.)

80. Finger Stroke Between the Eyebrows (Optional)

This technique relaxes the area between and just above the eyebrows and calms the mind.

Place your middle fingers between the eyebrows and then finger stroke up between the eyebrows a few times.

81. Finger Stroke Below the Eyebrows (Optional)

This technique relaxes the area under the eyebrows.

With your middle fingers, stroke under the recipient's eyebrows several times. (See photo 193 on page 238.)

82. Thumb Stroke down the Sides of the Nose (Optional)

This technique can help with nasal congestion.

With your thumbs, stroke down the sides of the recipient's nose. Your fingers will be under the jaw. (See photo 194 on page 238.)

83. Thumb Stroke below the Nose, above the Upper Lip

This technique relaxes the area between the nose and upper lip.

Place your thumbs below the recipient's nose and above the upper lip. With your thumbs, stroke outward in both directions simultaneously. (See photo 195 on page 238.)

84. Massage the Chin and Jaw (Optional)

This technique relaxes the chin and jaw.

Hold the recipient's chin between your thumbs and index fingers, with your fingers under the jaw. With a circling motion of your thumbs, massage from the chin outward along the jaw.

85. Massage the Jaw Muscles (Optional)

This technique relaxes the jaw and the masseter (major jaw) muscles.

With your fingertips, massage the jaw, working on the jaw muscles. (See photo 197 on page 239.)

86. Twist the Ears (Optional)

This technique relaxes the ears.

Twist the recipient's earlobes at various places. (See photo 198 on page 239.)

87. Relax the Eyes (Optional)

This technique relaxes the eyes.

Rub your palms together until they are hot. Then place your fingertips gently on the recipient's eyes.

Note: You should not perform this technique if the recipient is wearing contact lenses.

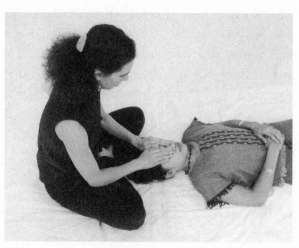

87. Relax the Eyes

10

THE TRADITIONAL SEQUENCE: THE SIDE-LYING POSITION

We can approach the importance of compassion through intelligent reasoning. If I help another person, and show concern for him or her, then I myself will benefit from that. However, if I harm others, eventually I will be in trouble.

—HIS HOLINESS THE DALAI LAMA

The basic side-lying position for a female is, first, on her left side with her left leg straight and her right leg bent. Her back should be straight and a pillow should be placed under her head. After completing the sequence, have her turn over and lie on her right side. Then repeat the sequence. A male should lie on his right side first and then on his left side.

This position is very useful for pregnant women and for people who cannot lie comfortably on their backs for long periods of time. The side-lying position is especially effective for shoulder and hip work. During the treatment, make sure to keep the recipient correctly aligned in this position—that is, with the spine straight, even if it means readjusting him or her during the treatment. Do the whole side-lying position on one side and then do the other side.

The Legs

88. Work on the Straight Leg

These techniques relax the intrinsic muscles on the sole of the foot, the calf muscles, and the muscles on the inner and back side of the straight leg, specifically the soleus, gastrocnemius, hamstring, and adductor muscles; and they stimulate the flow of energy there, which in turn relaxes and stimulates the flow of energy in the upper body. They also prepare the leg for the thumb press walking on the energy lines that follow. They are very grounding.

A. Knee and Palm Press on the Sole and Calf, Standard Version

This technique relaxes the intrinsic muscles on the sole of the foot and the calf muscles.

Assume a crawling position at the foot of the recipient's straight left leg. Place your right knee on the sole of the recipient's foot and your left hand on the recipient's calf. Then rock forward from your pelvis. Move your knee to another place on the foot and your hand to another place on the calf and rock forward again. Here, your knee and hand are pressing simultaneously. Repeat a few times.

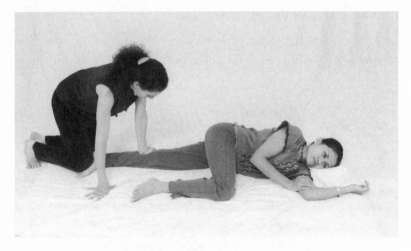

88A. Knee and Palm Press on the Sole and Calf of the Straight Leg

B. Knee Press on the Calf, Variation for Stronger Pressure (Optional)

This technique relaxes the calf and calf muscles, specifically the soleus and gastrocnemius muscles.

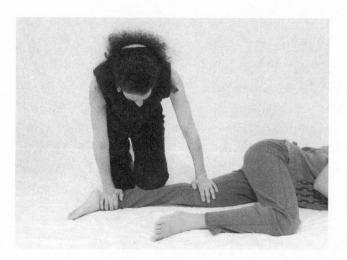

88B. Knee Press on the
Calf of the Straight Leg

Assume a crawling position facing the recipient's left leg. Place your right hand near the right ankle. Place your left hand on the right lower leg or on the mat between the recipient's legs. Place one of your knees on the recipient's calf and knee press up and down it.

Note: Knee pressing is stronger than palm pressing and can be used if the recipient's muscles are very hard.

C. Palm Press Walk Up the Straight Leg

Come to a crawling position behind the recipient's left leg. Invert your right hand and place it just above the ankle. Place your left hand just above the

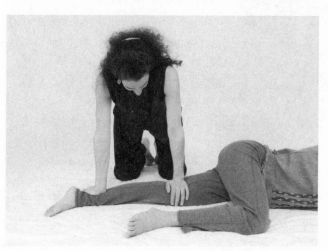

88C. Palm Press Walk Up
the Straight Leg

knee. Palm press walk up the leg, with your arms coming down at a ninety-degree angle. As you palm press, feel the condition of the leg.

D. Palm Press Walk Down the Straight Leg

After you reach the top of the lower leg with your right hand and the top of the thigh with your left hand, drop your hips and move your hands toward the back of the leg. Your right hand should no longer be inverted. Palm press walk down the leg with your arms coming in at a seventy-five-degree angle.

Repeat palm press walking up and then down the leg two more times.

INNER LEG LINES IN THE SIDE-LYING POSITION

Inner Leg Line 1 (side-lying) is the same as Inner Leg Line 1 in the supine position. (See page 88.) Inner Leg Line 2 (side-lying) is the same as Inner Leg Line 2 in the supine position. (See page 88.) Inner Leg Line 3 (side-lying) is the same as Inner Leg Line 3 in the supine position. (See page 88.) Inner Leg Line 4 (side-lying) runs in the middle of the thigh—*middle* here refers to how the thigh is exposed in the side-lying position.

The way the lines are worked in the side-lying position is different from how they are worked in the supine position due to the different way that the leg is exposed. For this reason, Inner Leg Line 2 is worked on the calf followed by work on Inner Leg Line 3 on the thigh. Similarly, Inner Leg Line 3 is worked on the calf followed by work on Inner Leg Line 4 on the thigh.

Note: Inner Leg Line 1 is not worked on in side-lying position. It is not visible in the drawing due to the angle that the drawing was done from.

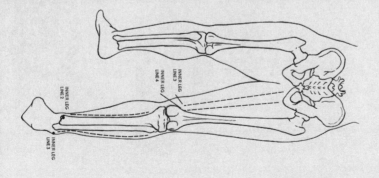

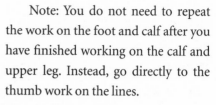

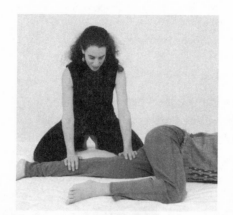

88D. Palm Press
Down the
Straight Leg

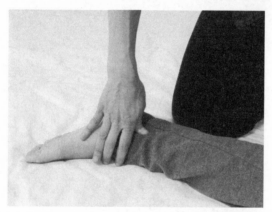

Note: You do not need to repeat the work on the foot and calf after you have finished working on the calf and upper leg. Instead, go directly to the thumb work on the lines.

89. Thumb Press Walk on Inner Leg Lines 2 and 3

This technique stimulates the flow of energy along Inner Leg Lines 2 and 3.

With your right thumb, thumb press on the starting point of Inner Leg Line 2. Thumb press walk up the lower leg, with your thumbs horizontally on Inner Leg Line 2. When you get to the knee area, slide your thumbs over it, tracing Inner Leg Line 2. Thumb press walk up the thigh with your thumbs horizontally on Inner Leg Line 3. Swivel your leading hand near the top of the thigh. Thumb press walk down the leg on

89. Thumb Press
Walk on Inner Leg
Lines 2 and 3

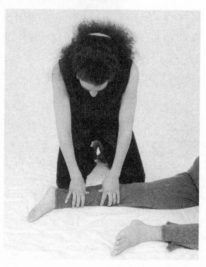

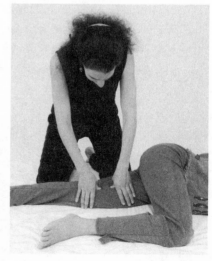

Inner Leg Lines 3 and 2 the same way you walked up them. Finish by pressing on the starting point of Inner Leg Line 2 with your right thumb.

90. Thumb Press Walk on Inner Leg Lines 3 and 4

This technique stimulates the flow of energy along Inner Leg Lines 3 and 4.

With crossed thumbs, thumb press on the starting point of Inner Leg Line 3. Then thumb press walk up the calf on Inner Leg Line 3 with your thumbs vertically crossing the line. Slide over the knee and then, with your thumbs horizontally on the line, thumb press walk up the thigh on Inner Leg Line 4. Swivel your leading hand near the top of the thigh. For more pressure, you can press with crossed thumbs at the top of the thigh. Thumb press walk down the leg on Inner Leg Lines 4 and 3 the same way you walked up them. Finish by pressing on the starting point of Inner Leg Line 3 with crossed thumbs.

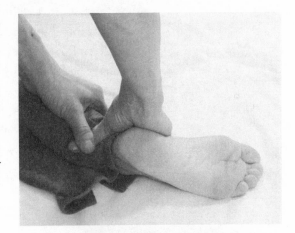

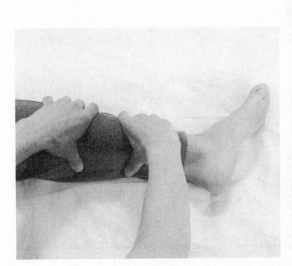

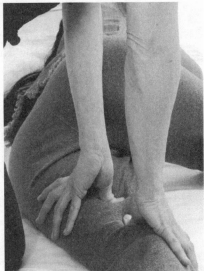

90. Thumb Press Walk on Inner Leg Lines 3 and 4

91. Stop the Blood on the Straight Leg

These techniques stop and release the blood.

The standard technique is to stop the blood in a seated position. However, if lighter pressure is desired, substitute one of the variations that follow the standard instructions.

A. Standard Procedure: Seated Position

Move the recipient's left leg out to the side a little. Sit down on your left buttock at the top of the thigh. Place both of your legs on the outside of the recipient's left leg. Have your left thigh resting on the left leg. Place your right foot on the heel of your left foot. Lean back so that your spine rests on the recipient's buttocks. Feel the person's femoral pulse through your buttock and stay there for sixty pulses. Then place your hands on the mat and very slowly raise yourself up a little, all the while keeping contact with the leg. Sit down again a little further down the leg and stay again for sixty pulses. Slowly raise yourself up a little and then sit down once more a little further down the thigh. Stay in this position for sixty pulses. Repeat this procedure going back up the thigh, staying at each place that you rest for sixty pulses. The full sequence is 1-2-3-2-1. It should take about five minutes.

Note: If the person you are working on has a very stiff lower back, you can stay even longer in each position—up to one hundred pulses at each place, but make sure that the recipient lets you know if he or she starts to feel uncomfortable.

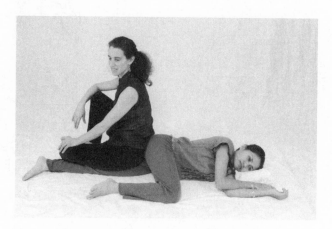

91A. Stop the Blood in
      a Seated Position

B. Variation 1 for Lighter Pressure: Stop the Blood with Your Hands

Come to a crawling position next to the recipient's left thigh. Place either one or both (for more pressure) of your hands on the thigh near the groin and lean. Feel for the pulse and then hold for sixty pulses. Release and then repeat four more times.

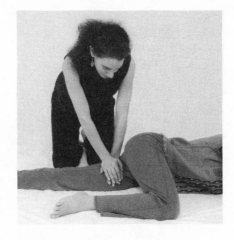

91B. Stop the Blood with Your Hand

C. Variation 2 for Medium Pressure: Stop the Blood with Your Knee

Come to a kneeling position with your right knee on the thigh near the groin and your left knee on the mat. Feel for the pulse and then hold for sixty pulses. Release and then repeat up to four more times.

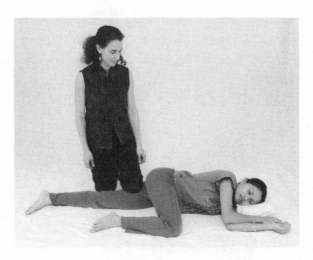

91C. Stop the Blood with Your Knee

92. Palm Press Walk on the Bent Leg

This technique relaxes the outside of the leg and the muscles there, specifically the iliotibial tract and the peroneus and quadriceps muscles.

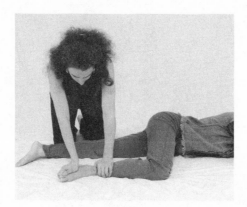

92A. Palm Press Walk on the Foot and Lower Leg

A. Palm Press Walk on the Foot and Lower Leg

Come to a kneeling position behind the recipient's left leg. Place your right hand, inverted, on the foot and your left hand, straight, on the lower leg just above the ankle. Palm press walk up the side of the foot and lower leg. Repeat going back down and then up.

B. Palm Press Walk on the Lower Leg and Thigh

Change to a half-lunge position so that your right knee is down on the mat between the recipient's legs and your left foot is at the side of the back. Place your right hand on the lower leg just above the ankle and your left hand on the thigh just above the knee. Palm press walk up the leg. Do not apply too much pressure on the upper leg as there is nothing supporting it. Apply your weight more to the lower leg, which is supported by the mat. Palm press walk down the leg. Repeat the palm press walking up and down the leg two more times.

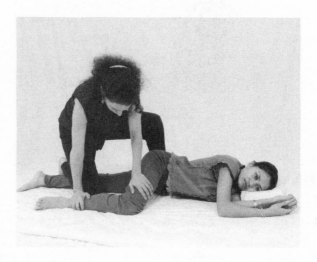

92B. Palm Press Walk on the Lower Leg and Thigh

OUTER LEG LINES IN THE SIDE-LYING POSITION

Outer Leg Line 1 (side-lying) runs at the same place as Outer Leg Line 1 in the supine position. (See page 94.)

Outer Leg Line 2 (side-lying) starts below the outer anklebone. On the lower leg, the line runs below the outer side of the fibula—not on the fibula as it did in supine. On the thigh, the line starts in the hollow above the tendon at the knee and then goes up the back of the thigh to the area between the top of the femur and the ischial tuberosity (the "sit bone").

Outer Leg Line 3 (side-lying) starts on the Achilles tendon. On the lower leg, the line runs up the middle of the calf at the same place as Outer and Inner Leg Line 3 (supine). On the thigh, the line runs from above the back of the knee to the ischial tuberosity.

Note: Outer Leg Line 1 is not worked on in the side-lying position. It is not shown in the drawing as it is not visible from the angle the drawing was done from.

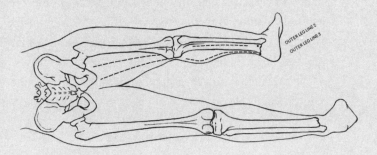

C. Palm Press Walk on the Lower Leg and Foot

Come back to the lower leg and foot. Change your legs back to the position in 92A and palm press down, up, and down again, finishing with your right hand at the end of the foot and your left hand at the bottom of the lower leg.

93. Thumb Press Walk on Outer Leg Line 2

This technique stimulates the flow of energy along Outer Leg Line 2.

Come to a half-kneeling, half-lunging position. With your right thumb, thumb press on the starting point of Outer Leg Line 2. On the lower

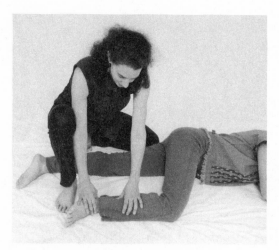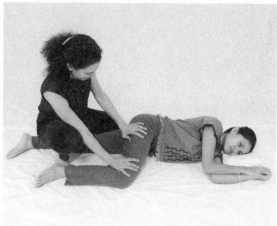

93. Thumb Press Walk on Outer Leg Line 2

leg, thumb press walk up just behind the fibula (the smaller of the two bones in the lower leg) on Outer Leg Line 2. Thumb press in the hollow above the tendon at the knee. On the thigh, thumb press walk up on Outer Leg Line 2. Go a little way up the buttock on Outer Leg Line 2 until you have reached the area between the greater trochanter (the prominence at the top of the thighbone) and the ischial tuberosity (the "sit bone"). Thumb press walk down the leg on Outer Leg Line 2 the same way you walked up it.

94. Thumb Press Walk on Outer Leg Line 3

This technique stimulates the flow of energy along Outer Leg Line 3.

With crossed thumbs, press on the Achilles tendon on the starting point of Outer Leg Line 3. With your thumbs vertical, thumb press walk up the lower leg on Outer Leg Line 3. On the thigh, thumb press walk up on Outer Leg Line 3 until you reach the ischial tuberosity (the "sit bone"). You can use your thigh as a lever to give strength to your thumb presses. Thumb press walk down the leg on Outer Leg Line 3 the same way you walked up it.

95. Bent Leg Straightened Out to the Side (Optional)

Pressure from your fingers on the front of the thigh stimulates the flow of energy along Inner Leg Line 1 and relaxes the quadriceps muscles. The outstretched position of the leg mobilizes the hip joint, stretches the hamstring

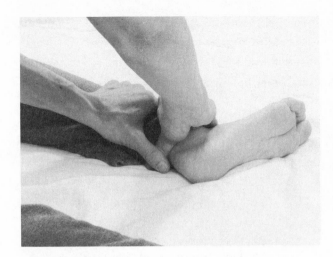

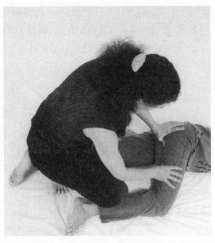

94. Thumb Press Walk on Outer Leg Line 3

muscles, and stimulates the flow of energy along Outer Leg Lines 2 and 3. The spinal twist at the end increases spinal mobility.

A. Pull the Front of the Thigh

Kneel on your left knee, and be up on the ball of your left foot. Place the recipient's right ankle between your right big toe and your second toe. Place your left hand above the knee as a support and then move your right foot out to the side, bringing the leg with you until it is straight and has gone as

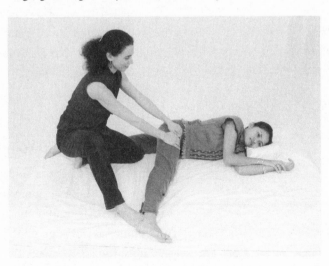

95A. Pull the Front of the Thigh

far as it can comfortably go. Place both of your hands on the top of the thigh. Pull the leg toward you. Move your hands to the middle of the thigh and repeat. Move your hands down to just above the knee and repeat. Go up and down the thigh several times, pulling it toward you with your fingers.

B. Knee Press on the Back of the Thigh

Place your left knee on the back of the recipient's thigh and your hands on the opposite side on the front of the thigh. Press in with your knee as you pull the thigh toward you with your hands. Repeat the simultaneous pressing and pulling up and down the thigh.

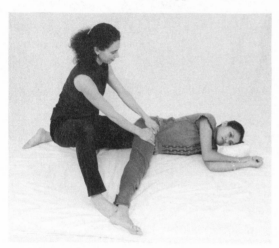

95B. Knee Press on the Back of the Thigh

C. Thumb Press Outer Leg Lines 2 and 3

Return to the kneeling position described in Step 95A. Thumb press walk down the thigh and lower leg on Outer Leg Line 2. With crossed thumbs, press the starting point of Outer Leg Line 3. Thumb press walk up the calf on Outer Leg Line 3. Thumb press walk up the thigh on Outer Leg Line 2.

D. Spinal Twist

With your left hand, bring the recipient's right arm back. Then put your left hand on the shoulder and your right hand on the lower leg and press down on the shoulder.

The Hip and Buttock

96. One Leg Back (Optional)

This position stretches the iliopsoas (the muscle that attaches the lower spine to the legs) and quadriceps muscles and mobilizes the hip joint. The abdominal work relaxes the abdominal organs and stimulates peristalsis.

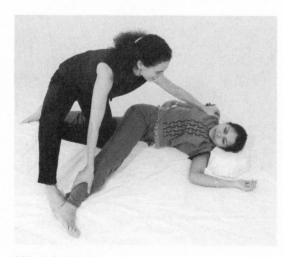

95D. Spinal Twist

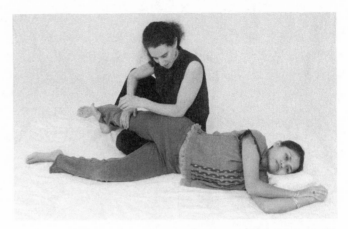

96A. Work the Hip with One Leg Back

A. Elbow Press on the Hip

Sit behind the recipient's legs. Swing the right leg back toward you and bring your right leg out to the side. Have your right heel down and your toes up. Place the leg over your ankle, holding it in place that way. Lean in on the hip with your left elbow. Work around the hip at a few places.

B. Elbow Press on the Abdomen

Work with your left elbow at various places on the abdomen by placing your elbow on the abdomen and leaning in.

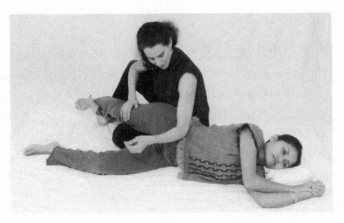

96B. Elbow Press on the Abdomen with One Leg Back

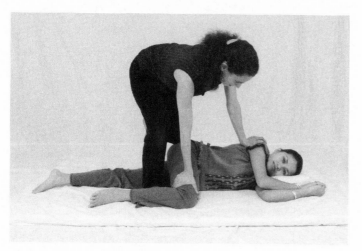

97. Knee Press on the Buttock

97. Knee Press on the Buttock (Optional)

This technique using knee pressure, which is more powerful than other types of pressure, is very effective for relaxing the buttocks and helps sciatica. The gluteus (buttock) muscles are relaxed.

With your left hand, hold the recipient's right shoulder, and with your right hand, hold the leg to steady yourself. Place your right foot between the recipient's legs. With your left knee, press on the buttock.

The Back

98. Thumb Press on the Waistline

This technique acquaints you with the waist and begins to relax it.

Come to a half-lunge position, with your right knee down and your left knee up, with your left foot near the recipient's back. Face the recipient's head. Place your right hand on the hip and your left hand, with the thumb pointing up, on the waist and press down with your thumb. Both of your arms should be straight. Move your left thumb down and press again. Repeat a few times.

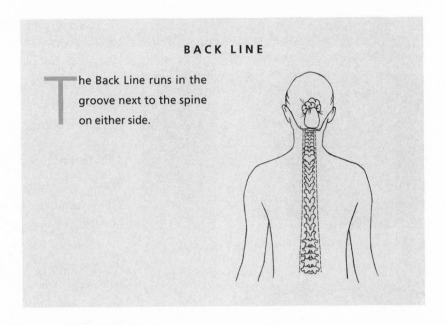

BACK LINE

The Back Line runs in the groove next to the spine on either side.

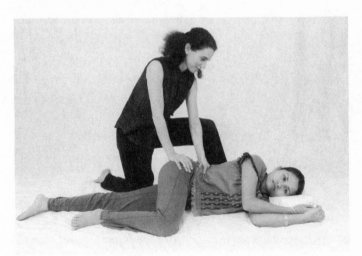

98. Thumb Press on the Waistline

99. Thumb Press Walk along the Back Line Above the Spine

This technique stimulates the flow of energy along the Back Line and relaxes the back muscles, specifically the erector spinae, trapezius, latissimus dorsi, and rhomboid muscles.

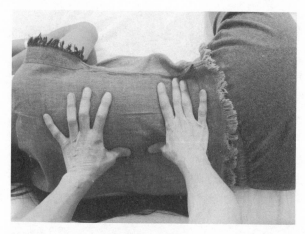

99. Thumb Press Walk along the Back Line Above the Spine

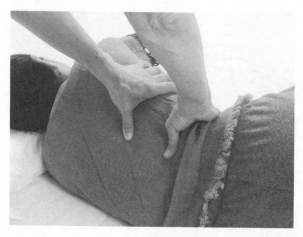

100. Thumb Press Down toward the Spine

Change your position so that you are kneeling with your knees spread open facing the recipient's back. Thumb press walk up and down the back line with your thumbs horizontally on the Back Line above the spine. Repeat two more times.

100. Thumb Press Down toward the Spine

This technique increases the side-to-side mobilization of the spine.

Push the recipient forward a little so that the back is no longer so vertical. This will make it easier for you to do the following techniques without hyperextending your wrists. Place your thumbs facing down just above the spine and then press downward. As you press down, rock forward from your pelvis to increase the pressure. Go up and down along the spine while continuing to rock forward. Repeat two times.

101. Thumb Roll

This technique relaxes the back.

A. Over Upper Erectors

Place your thumbs on the lower back in the groove between the spine and the upper erector spinae muscles (the muscles that run by the side of the spine). Then roll up over the erector spinae muscles. In this way, continue up the back as far as you can while still rolling over the muscle. When you can no longer roll over the muscle, go back down the back in the same way. Repeat several times.

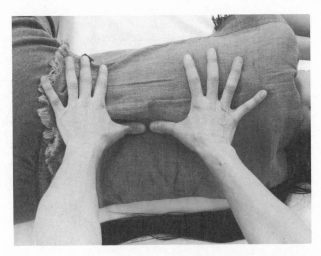

101A. Thumb Roll over Upper Erectors

B. Over Lower Erectors

Place your thumbs below the lower erector spinae muscles and then roll up over them. In this way, continue up and down the back. Repeat several times.

Note: The area of the back where you roll up over the erector spinae muscles is determined by where you can effectively do the rolling movement.

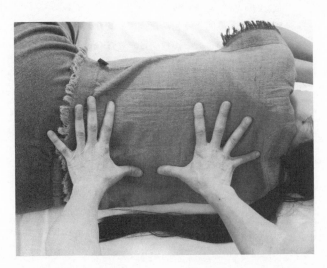

101B. Thumb Roll over Lower Erectors

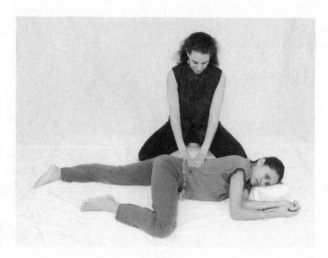

102. Squeeze the
Lower Back

102. Squeeze the Lower Back

This technique relaxes the lower back, specifically the erector spinae and latissimus dorsi muscles.

Place your hands on the recipient's lumbar (lower) back with your fingers and thumbs spread apart.

Squeeze the lower back between your thumbs and fingers. Make sure to use equal pressure with your thumbs and fingers. Squeeze up and down the lumbar back a few times.

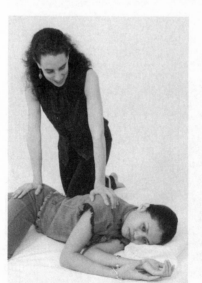

103A. Knee Press on
the Lower Back with
One Knee

103. Knee Press on the Lower Back (Optional)

This technique relaxes the lower back, specifically the latissimus dorsi and erector spinae muscles.

A. With One Knee

Place your right hand on the recipient's hip and your left hand on the shoulder. Then place one of your knees on the lumbar back below the spine. Slowly increase the weight on your knee by rocking forward from your pelvis. Repeat with your knee at other places on the lumbar and lower thoracic back (the chest portion of the back).

B. With Both Knees

Knee press walk with one knee after the other on the lumbar and lower thoracic back.

The Shoulder Blade

This technique loosens up the shoulder blade and the surrounding area, specifically the levator scapula, rhomboid, and trapezius muscles.

104. Thumb Press Around the Shoulder Blade

A. Upper Part of the Shoulder Blade

Sit down facing the recipient's back with your left leg bent and your right leg extended. If the recipient's back is not vertical, bring it back toward you so that it is. Place the right arm behind the back (this will make it easier to work around the shoulder blade). Place your left thumb by the upper inner border of the shoulder blade and your right hand on the shoulder. Pull the shoulder back toward you a little as you press up under the shoulder blade with your thumb. Use your left leg as a brace for your left arm as you do the thumb pressing. In this way, work around the upper inside border of the shoulder blade.

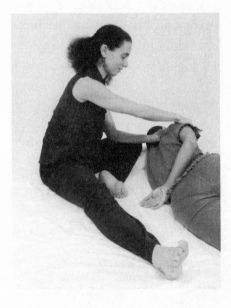

104A. Thumb Press Around the Upper Part of the Shoulder Blade

B. Lower Part of the Shoulder Blade

Change the position of your hands so that your right thumb is by the lower inner side of the shoulder blade and your left hand is on the shoulder. Bend your right leg and have your knee work as a brace for your right arm. Pull the shoulder back toward you a little as you press up under the shoulder blade with your thumb. Use your knee to support your arm as you do the thumb pressing. In this way, work around the lower inner border of the shoulder blade.

105. Toes Under the Shoulder Blade (Optional)

These techniques loosen the shoulder blade, expand the chest, relax the back, and mobilize the spine.

A. One Foot

Sit down behind the recipient's back and hold the right arm at the shoulder and elbow. Place the toes of your left foot by the inner border of the right shoulder blade. Bring the arm back toward you and hold the right hand with your right hand. Hold the wrist or forearm with your left hand. Pull the arm toward you so that the shoulder blade rolls over your toes. Do not press in with your toes. Release the pull. Move your toes to another place by the shoulder blade and pull the arm again. Repeat this movement several times with your toes at different places by the shoulder blade.

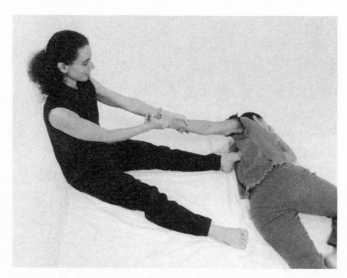

105A. Toes Under the Shoulder Blade: One Foot

B. Two Feet

Place the toes of both of your feet by the inside border of the shoulder blade and pull the arm so that the shoulder blade rolls over your toes toward you. Repeat a few times at different places.

C. Two Feet on the Back

Place the balls of both of your feet on the recipient's back. Pull the arm toward you. Repeat with your feet at other places on the back.

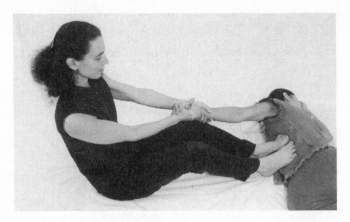

105C. Two Feet on the Back

D. Heel on the Hip

Move forward a little. Place the toes of your left foot by the right shoulder blade. Place your right heel by the recipient's right hip. Pull the arm back

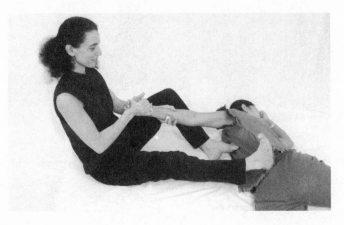

105D. Heel on the Hip

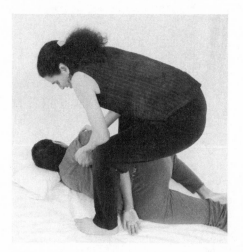

106. Shoulder-Blade Lift

toward you so that the shoulder blade rolls over your toes as you simultaneously push the hip forward with your heel. Repeat a few times with your heel at different places on the hip.

106. Shoulder-Blade Lift (Optional)

This technique mobilizes the shoulder blade.

Bend the right arm at the elbow and place it behind the recipient's back. Step over the recipient and face the head. With your right hand, hold the front of the shoulder. With the fingertips of your left hand, hook the inner border of the shoulder blade. Lift the recipient up. Repeat a few times.

The Arm and Hand

107. Palm Press Walk on the Back of the Arm

This technique relaxes the arm and compresses all of the back arm muscles. It is very grounding.

Place the arm on the side of the recipient's body, with the palm facing down. Come to a half-lunge position with your left knee down on the mat

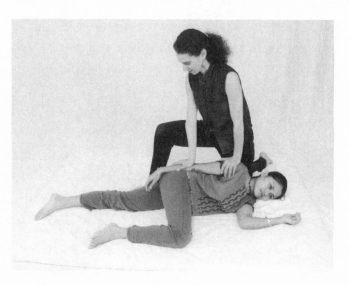

107. Palm Press Walk on the Back of the Arm

BACK ARM LINE IN THE SIDE-LYING POSITION

The Back Arm Line (side-lying) starts just above the outer side of the wrist. On the forearm, it runs on the outer side between the radius and ulna (the two forearm bones). On the upper arm, it runs behind the humerus to the top of the arm.

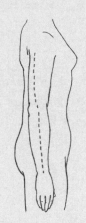

and your right knee up. Your left knee should support the recipient's back and shoulder. Place your left hand at the top of the arm and your right hand just below the elbow. In this way, hold the arm between your hands. Palm press walk down the arm. Keep your arms straight and let all of your body weight go through your arms. Palm press walk back up the arm. Palm press walk down the arm again so that you end up with your right hand by the recipient's wrist and your left hand by the elbow.

108. Thumb Press Walk on the Back Arm Line

This technique stimulates the flow of energy along the Back Arm Line.

Come to a kneeling position, with your knees open and your

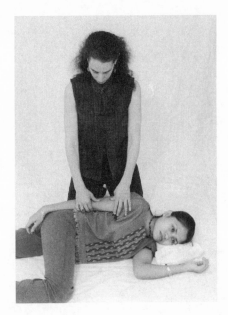

108. Thumb Press Walk on the Back Arm Line

FRONT ARM LINE IN THE
SIDE-LYING POSITION

The Front Arm Line (side-lying) starts just above the inner side of the wrist. On the forearm, it runs in the middle of the inner side. On the upper arm, it runs on top of the triceps.

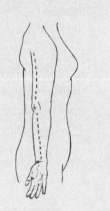

hips up. Hold the recipient's arm with your fingers and place your thumbs horizontally on the line above the wrist. Thumb press walk up and down the Back Arm Line. Repeat one time.

Note: As you thumb press walk on the back of the arm, make sure to keep your fingertips on the arm so that there is contact from both your thumbs and your fingers.

109. Thumb Press Walk on the Front Arm Line

This technique stimulates the flow of energy along the Front Arm Line.

Drop your hips down so that you are sitting on your heels. Spread your knees open. Turn the recipient's arm so that the palm faces you and rest the forearm on the buttock. Clasp the arm between

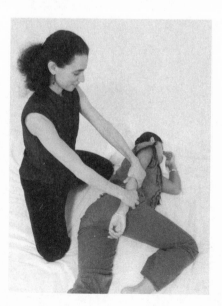

109. Thumb Press Walk on the Front Arm Line

your hands with your thumbs placed vertically across the line. Thumb press walk up the Front Arm Line. Then thumb press walk down the arm. Repeat one time.

Note: As you thumb press walk on the front of the arm, also press on the back surface of the arm with your fingers so that both sides of the arm are pressed.

110. Thumb Press on Five Lines on the Palm

This technique stimulates Sen Kalathari, relaxes the intrinsic muscles and nerves on the palms, and affects the reflex points on the palms, which affect the corresponding areas of the body. (See page 138.)

Come to a kneeling position, facing the recipient's head, by the side of the left leg. Interlace your fingers from above with the recipient's fingers as follows:

- Slide your right pinkie between the recipient's middle and ring finger.

- Slide your right ring finger between the ring finger and pinkie.

- Slide your left pinkie between the recipient's middle and index finger.

- Slide your left ring and middle finger between the index finger and thumb.

This leaves the recipient's middle finger free. Thumb press with both of your thumbs simultaneously from the heel of the hand down to the thumb and pinkie. As you thumb press, press the hand against the buttock. Then thumb press down the palm to the index and ring finger. Lastly, thumb press with both of your thumbs to the middle finger. Repeat the thumb pressing down the palm a few more times. (See photo 63 on page 139.)

111. Finger Traction

This technique helps mobilize the finger joints.

Turn the recipient's arm so that the palm is facing down. With your left hand, hold the wrist. Interlace the fingers of your right hand with the recipient's fingers. With your fingers, press the fingers backward and then pull

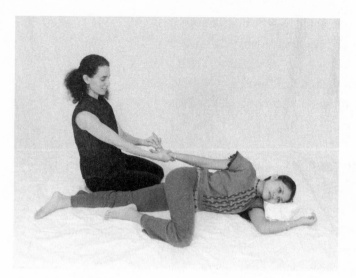

111. Finger Traction

them toward you. Slide your fingers up the fingers a little way. Once again press the fingers backward and then pull them toward you.

112. Rotate, Pull, and Crack the Fingers

This technique helps to mobilize the finger joints and helps bring wind (energy) to the fingers.

With your right hand, "hand-shake" the recipient's right hand and hold the knuckle above the pinkie between your thumb and index finger. With your left hand, hold the pinkie at the end between your index and middle finger with your fingers bent. Rotate the pinkie a few times in large circles to loosen it up as you simultaneously circle with your right thumb on the knuckle. Move your

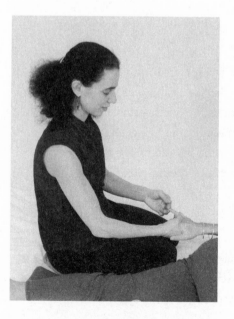

112. Rotate, Pull, and Crack the Fingers

index and middle finger to the base of the pinkie. Then pull back quickly. You will probably hear a cracking sound. If not, you can either try again or move on to the next finger. Repeat this procedure with each of the recipient's fingers, moving from the pinkie to the index finger.

Then release the handshake hold and hold the recipient's right hand near the thumb with your left thumb and index finger. Rotate the thumb between your right index and middle finger and then quickly pull the thumb.

Note: Do not perform this technique on anyone who has rheumatoid arthritis.

113. Massage the Fingers

This technique relaxes the fingers and stimulates circulation to the fingers.

Continue to hold the recipient's hand with your left hand. Hold just above the finger that you are working on. With your other hand, massage each finger by squeezing and sliding down it. Go from the thumb to the pinkie.

114. Stretch the Fingers Back

This technique mobilizes the fingers.

Hold the recipient's pinkie and thumb between your thumb and other fingers. Then stretch those fingers backward. Repeat with the index and ring finger and finish with the middle finger.

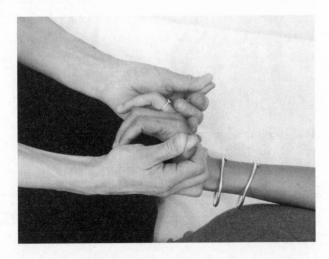

114. Stretch the Fingers Back

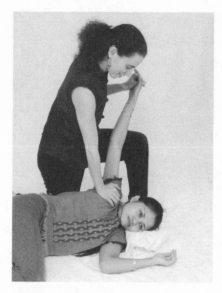 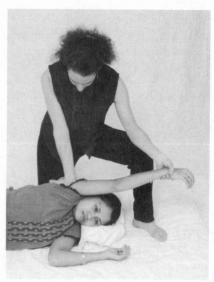

115. Palm Press on the Chest with the
Arm Up

116. Inverted Palm Press with the
Arm Overhead

115. Palm Press on the Chest with the Arm Up

This technique mobilizes the shoulder joint and relaxes the chest, specifically the pectoralis major muscle.

Interlace the fingers of your left hand with those of the recipient's right hand. Bring the arm in an arc in front of the body and then up above the body as you simultaneously raise your hips up and move forward to a half-lunge position with your left knee up and your right knee down on the mat supporting the recipient's body, which should be brought back toward you a little. Depending on the recipient's flexibility, either rest his or her arm on your left leg or hold it up. Place your right hand on the recipient's chest near the armpit. Lean in. Repeat a few times at different places.

116. Inverted Palm Press with the Arm Overhead

This technique helps to mobilize and relax the shoulder complex.

Bring the recipient's arm down by his or her side and then in an arc in front of the body over the head. Then hold it at the wrist. Turn so that you are facing the recipient's body. Invert your right hand and palm press on the side of the body just below the arm.

117. Stretch Arm Up (Optional)

This technique increases the range of motion of the shoulder complex and opens the chest, stretching the pectoralis major muscle.

Kneel behind the recipient's back with your hips up. With both of your hands, hold the recipient's arm at the wrist and bring it up. Then lean back a little, bringing the arm with you.

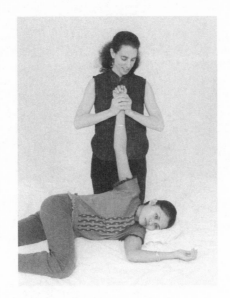

117. Stretch Arm Up

118. Side Stretch (Optional)

This technique stretches the side of the body.

Come to the head of the recipient in a half-lunge position with your right knee down near the back and your left knee up by the recipient's head. Place the right arm on your left thigh with the palm facing down. With your left hand, hold the forearm. Place your right hand on the hip. Push the hip away from you as you lean the other way.

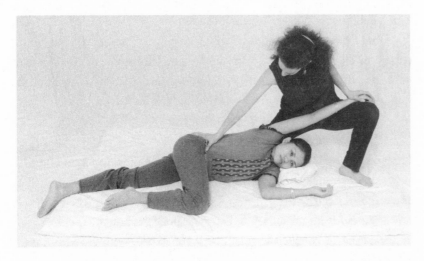

118. Side Stretch

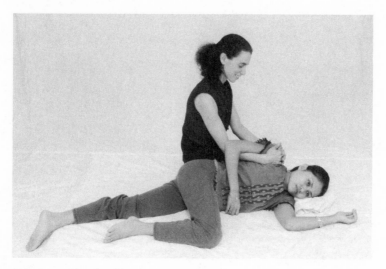

119. Rotate the Shoulder

119. Rotate the Shoulder (Optional)

This technique mobilizes the shoulder complex.

Kneel by the side of the recipient facing his or her head. Hold the recipient's shoulder between your hands with your fingers interlaced. The recipient's right arm should be over your right arm. Rotate the shoulder a few times.

120. Pull the Shoulder Back

This technique mobilizes the shoulder complex.

Hold the recipient's shoulder with your fingers interlaced. The arm can remain in the same position as in the previous technique or you can place the recipient's arm by the left side of your waist. Lean back and pull the shoulder toward the buttocks. Repeat the pulling back a few times.

121. Thumb Press Walk on the Front Arm Line

This technique stimulates the flow of energy along the Front Arm Line.

Come to a half-kneeling, half-lunging position with your right knee down and your left knee up. Bring the recipient's right arm out behind. Make sure not to bring it too far back, as that can cause strain on the shoulder joint. Rest the arm on your left leg just below your knee. With crossed thumbs,

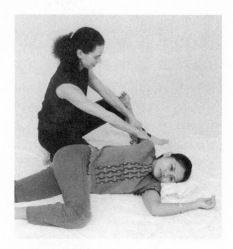

121. Thumb Press Walk on the Front Arm Line

press into the armpit. Then, with your thumbs pointing down, crossing the Front Arm Line, thumb press walk from the armpit to the wrist and back two times. As you thumb press walk, keep your arms stretched out.

122. Elbow Press on the Chest (Optional)

This technique mobilizes the shoulder complex, energizes the lungs, and relaxes the chest, specifically the pectoralis major muscle.

Kneel by the side of the recipient's back. Bring the recipient's arm back and rest it on your thighs. Hold the arm with your left hand. Place your right elbow on the side of the person's chest on the pectoralis major muscle. Press down with your elbow for a few seconds. Move your elbow to another place on the side of the chest and press again. Repeat a few times.

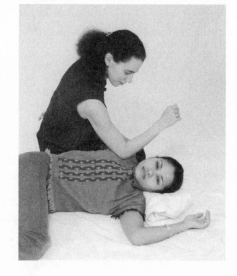

122. Elbow Press on the Chest

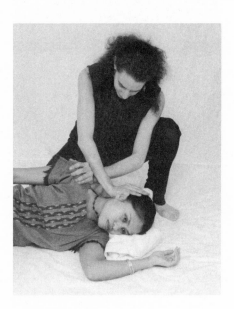

123. Crossed Arm
Neck Stretch

The Neck

123. Crossed Arm Neck Stretch (Optional)

This technique stretches the neck and helps to elongate shortened tissue between the base of the skull and the shoulder complex.

Half kneel and half lunge with your right knee down and your left knee up facing the recipient's neck from the back. Place your left hand on the recipient's shoulder and the heel of your right hand at the base of the skull. Press your hands in opposite directions.

Torso

124. Spinal Twist from Behind

This technique increases spinal mobility and stretches multiple tissues in the back.

Come to a half-lunge position behind the recipient. Make sure the back is vertical. Bring the recipient's arm out to the side and place the recipient's wrist on your left lower leg. Place your right hand on the thigh just above the knee. Place your left hand on the shoulder. Press down on the thigh as you simultaneously press down on the shoulder. As you press, rock forward from

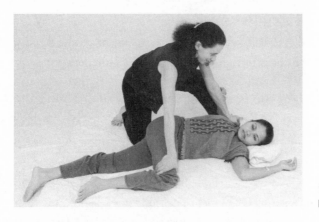

124. Spinal Twist from Behind

your pelvis. Move your right hand to the middle of the thigh, and once again simultaneously press down on the thigh and shoulder as you rock forward from your pelvis. Move your right hand to the back of the buttock and again press the buttock and shoulder down while rocking forward from your pelvis.

125. Spinal Twist from the Front (Optional)

This technique increases spinal mobility and stretches multiple tissues in the back.

A. With Your Hand

Kneel in front of the recipient. Place your right hand on the shoulder and your left hand on the buttock. Pull the buttock toward you as you simultaneously push the shoulder back down toward the mat.

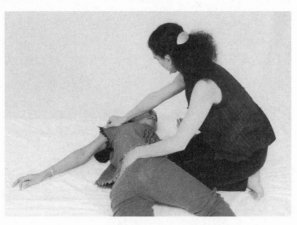

125. Spinal Twist from the Front, With Your Hand

B. With Your Elbow

Place your left elbow on the recipient's buttock. Press the buttock toward you as your right hand pushes the shoulder away from you toward the mat.

126. Pull Up the Bottom Leg while Holding the Top Arm

This technique increases the range of motion of the hip joint and stretches the abdominal, iliopsoas and front thigh muscles, specifically the quadriceps muscles.

Move the recipient's bent right leg down the mat a little so that it is no longer in such a bent position. Stand behind the recipient and pick up the right hand. Place it either on your left knee or hold it in the air. Simultaneously pick up the left ankle and pull the leg up toward you as you place your left foot on the sacrum. The pull should not be too strong. Lower the leg a little and then move your foot onto the lumbar (lower) back. Pull the leg up again. This pull should be medium in force. Lower the leg again a little and move your foot further up the lumbar back. Pull the leg up again. This pull should be the strongest. Repeat in the reverse. The full pattern is 1-2-3-2-1.

Bring the recipient back into the side-lying position.

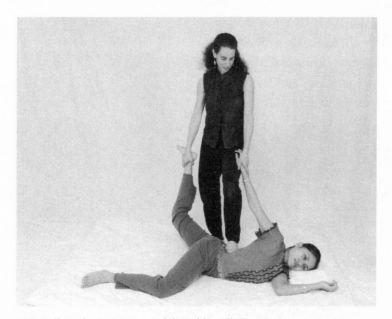

126. Pull Up the Bottom Leg while Holding the Top Arm

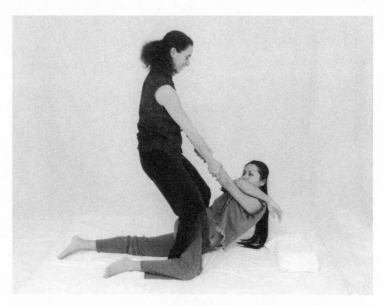

127. Spinal Twist While Pulling the Arm Up

127. Spinal Twist while Pulling the Arm Up

This technique mobilizes the shoulder complex and the spine and associated tissues.

Stand with your right leg behind the recipient's right bent leg and with your left leg by the side of the back. Drape the right arm over the left arm. With your left hand, hold the left hand, and with your right hand, hold the left forearm. Bend your knees and then pull the recipient up toward you. Lower the recipient. Move your left foot down toward you a little and then pull the recipient up again. Lower the recipient. Once again move your left foot down toward you a little and pull the recipient up again. Lower the recipient to the mat.

Note: Do not perform this technique on anyone who has osteoporosis or who has undergone a laminectomy or lumbar fusion surgery.

128. Arch the Recipient Back (Optional)

This technique improves the extension of the spine and stretches the abdomen, chest, and thigh, specifically the quadriceps, iliopsoas, rectus abdominis, and pectoralis major muscles.

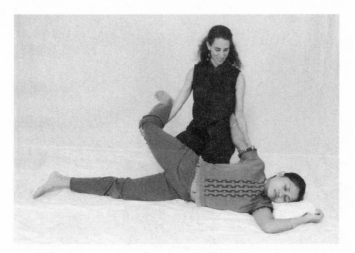

128. Arch the Recipient Back

Kneel behind the recipient. Place your left knee on the lumbar (lower) back and your right knee on the back of the right thigh. Place your left hand on the shoulder and slide your right hand under the right knee. Bring the leg back toward you. The recipient's body will remain stable due to the presence of your knees. As you pull the recipient's body back toward you, knee press up and down the back of the right thigh. To increase the stretch, place the recipient's right arm back by your waist. You can also bring your left hand to the front of the thigh and pull the leg toward you with your finger-

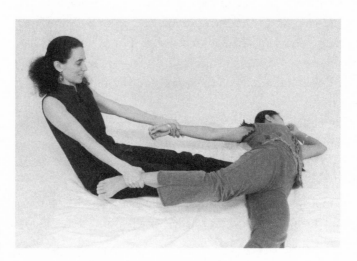

129. Both Feet on
        the Back

tips. Lastly, you can hold the front of the leg with both of your hands and pull the leg back toward you with your fingertips. Or you can pull the leg back toward you with one hand after the other as you walk your hands on the thigh.

129. Both Feet on the Back (Optional)

This technique improves the extension of the spine and stretches the front of the thigh, abdomen, and chest, specifically the quadriceps, iliopsoas, rectus abdominis, and pectoralis major muscles.

Sit behind the recipient's back. Bring the right arm and right leg back toward you and hold them. Place both of your feet on the back. Press your feet in as you pull the arm and leg toward you.

Once you have completed techniques 88 through 129 on one side of the recipient's body, repeat the entire side-lying sequence on the other side.

THE TRADITIONAL SEQUENCE: THE PRONE POSITION

As I mentioned before, genuine compassion is based on the recognition that others have the same right to happiness just like yourself, and therefore even your enemy is a human being with the same wish for happiness just like yourself and the same right to happiness as you. A sense of concern developed on this basis is what we call compassion; it extends to everyone irrespective of whether the person's attitude toward you is hostile or friendly.

—His Holiness The Dalai Lama

The basic prone position is on the stomach with the head turned to whichever side is more comfortable. The feet are rotated inward, with the toes facing in.

From time to time, have the recipient turn his or her head to the other side so as to not get a stiff neck. For people whose ankles do not rest on the mat, it is a good idea to put a rolled-up towel under each ankle after you have started the work on the buttocks.

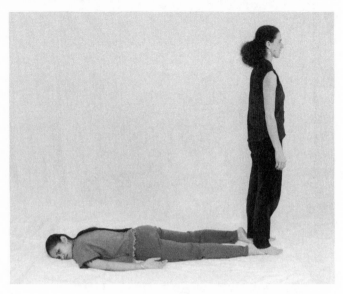

130. Walk on the Feet

130. Walk on the Feet

This technique is very grounding and relaxes the feet.

Stand on the recipient's feet facing away from the head. Walk up and down the soles of the feet, not including the heels.

131. Walk on One Foot (Optional)

This technique relaxes the arch of the foot.

Face the recipient's head. Stand on one of the feet with one of your feet, and with your other foot turned at an angle, press the inner side of the foot with the outer side of your foot. Then repeat the procedure on the other foot.

132. Palm Press Walk on the Legs

This technique relaxes and energizes the legs and compresses the hamstring and calf muscles, specifically the gastrocnemius and soleus muscles.

Turn around and face the recipient. Hold the ankles and pick up the legs. Rotate the feet outward and then place them down on the mat so that the toes point out. Kneel between the recipient's feet and palm press walk

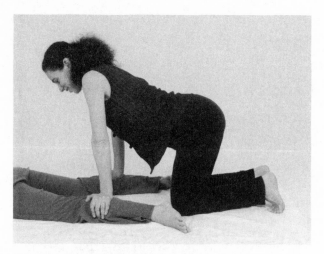

132. Palm Press Walk on the Legs

your hands alternately up the legs. As you walk up the lower legs, wrap the leg muscles in toward you before you press down on the fibula with the heels of your hands. Do not walk on the back of the knees. After you have reached the top of the legs, palm press walk down. Repeat two more times.

133. Thumb Press Walk on the Back Leg Lines

This technique stimulates the flow of energy along Back Leg Lines 2, 3, and 4.

Thumb press behind the outer anklebones at the starting point of Leg Line 2 on both ankles simultaneously. Thumb press walk up the calves behind the fibulas on Leg Line 2. Walk one thumb after the other on opposite legs. Continue up the thighs on Leg Line 3. Thumb press on both ischial tuberosities (the "sit bones") simultaneously. Thumb press walk down the thighs further in, on Leg Line 4. Continue down the middle of the backs of the calves on Leg Line 3. Thumb press on both Achilles tendons simultaneously.

Repeat the thumbing up and down the legs two more times.

Note: You are making a loop each time you thumb press up and down the lines in the prone position.

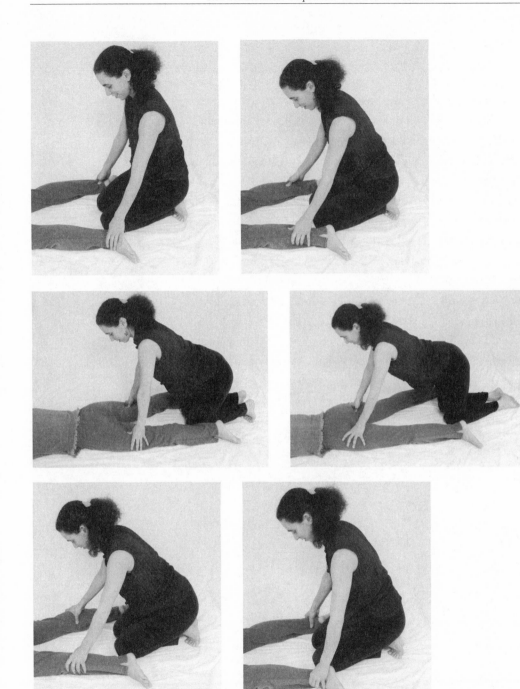

133. Thumb Press Walk on the Leg Lines on the Back of the Legs

BACK LEG LINES IN THE PRONE POSITION

There is no Leg Line 1 in the prone position.

Back Leg Line 2 (prone) starts behind the outer anklebone, and then runs behind the fibula, in the same place on the lower leg as Outer Leg Line 2 in the side-lying position. The thigh portion is not worked on.

Back Leg Line 3 (prone) starts on the Achilles tendon and then runs along the middle of the posterior calf to the back of the knee. From the knee, it goes up to the ischial tuberosity (the "sit bone").

Back Leg Line 4 (prone) runs on the thigh only, and runs to the inside of Outer Leg Line 3.

Note: In the prone position, thumb press walk up Back Leg Line 2 on the lower legs and then Back Leg Line 3 on the thighs up to the ischial tuberosity. Thumb press walk down Leg Line 4 on the thighs and then down Back Leg Line 3 on the lower legs. You will be making a loop as you thumb press up and down the leg lines.

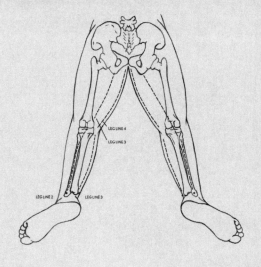

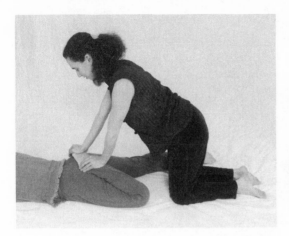
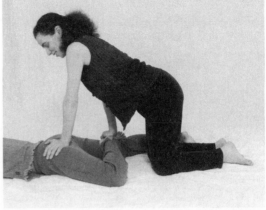

134. Bend the Leg Back and Press the Foot to the Buttock

135. Palm Press on the Buttock and Bent Leg

134. Bend the Leg Back and Press the Foot to the Buttocks

This technique mobilizes the knee and ankle joints and stretches the front of the thigh.

Hold the recipient's left foot with both of your hands and bend the leg back. Then press the foot toward the buttocks.

135. Palm Press on the Buttock and Bent Leg

This technique mobilizes the knee joint, softens buttock muscles, enhances the function of the sciatic nerve, and relaxes the hamstring muscles.

Place the recipient's left ankle on the back of the thigh of the straight leg above the back of the right knee. Hold the left foot in place with your right hand, and with your left hand palm press on the left buttock and down the back of the left thigh. Then go back up and down again. Both of your arms should be straight as you do this.

136. Knee Press on the Bent Leg

This technique increases the range of motion of the hip and knee joints, stimulates the flow of energy along Outer Leg Line 1 (supine), and relaxes the tibialis anterior muscle, the muscle adjacent to the shinbone.

Move the recipient's left foot further up on the back of the right thigh.

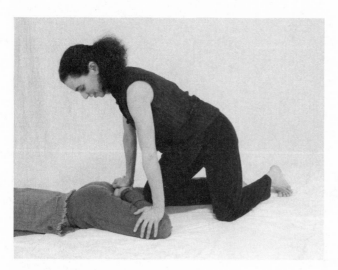

136. Knee Press on the Bent Leg

Place your left hand on the recipient's thigh just above the knee and keep your right hand on the foot. Place one of your knees on the muscle above the tibia (the shinbone) and lean forward. In this way, knee press above the shinbone on the upper and middle section of the lower leg several times. Do not knee press on the area directly above the ankle.

Once you have completed techniques 134 through 136 on one side of the recipient's body, repeat the sequence on the other side.

137. Crossed Feet Press

This technique stimulates the reflex areas on the soles of the feet and increases the range of motion of the ankle and knee joints.

Bend the recipient's legs at the knees and cross the feet so that the top of one foot is over the other. With your hands, press the feet toward the buttocks. Exchange the position of the feet and press them toward the buttocks again.

Note: Do not perform this technique on anyone who has a history of disk problems, as it compresses the lower back.

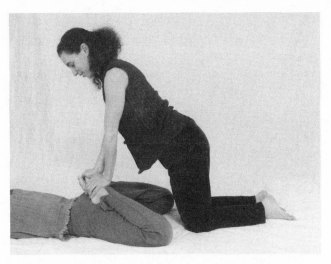

137. Crossed Feet Press

138. Sit on the Back (Optional)

A. Knee Walk on the Calves

This technique relaxes the calves, specifically the gastrocnemius and soleus muscles.

Sit on the recipient's lumbar (lower) back or sacrum facing the feet. Hold the ankles. Place your knees on the calves and walk them up and down the calves. Simultaneously assist the movement with your hands by moving

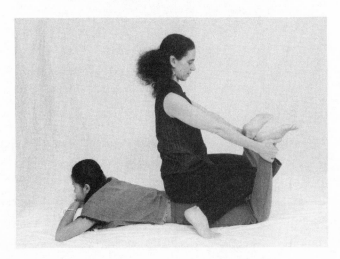

138A. Knee Walk on the Calves While Sitting on the Back

the legs back and forth a little so that you can walk your knees up and down the calves. Walk with the outer side of your knees.

B. Lean Back While Pulling the Legs Back

This technique mobilizes the lower region of the spine, rotates the pelvis, and stretches the iliopsoas (the muscle that connects the lumbar spine to the thighbone) and quadriceps muscles.

Place your knees on the recipient's Achilles tendons. Continue to hold the legs at the ankles. Raise your heels as you lean back, pulling the recipient's legs toward you. Your arms should be straight as you lean back. Lower your heels as you let the recipient's legs down. Move up the back slightly. Raise your heels again as you lean back further, pulling the recipient's legs toward you. Lower your heels as you let the recipient's legs down again. Move up the back a bit further. Raise your heels again as you lean back even further, pulling the recipient's legs toward you. Lower your heels to the mat and lower the recipient's legs.

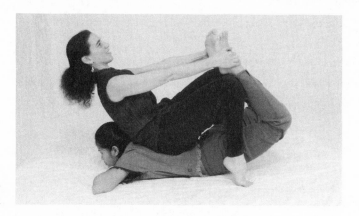

138B. Lean Back While Pulling the Legs Back

139. Crossed Leg Pull-Up

This technique increases the mobility of the hip joint; extends the lower regions of the spine, making it more flexible; and stretches the iliopsoas and quadriceps muscles.

Bend the recipient's right leg at the knee and place the right foot behind the left knee. Then stand by the right side near the lumbar (lower) back. Hold the recipient's left leg just above the ankle with your left hand. Place

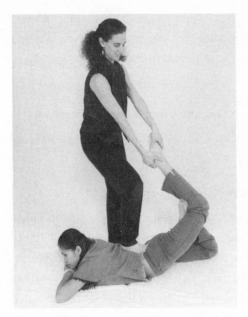

139. Crossed Leg Pull-Up

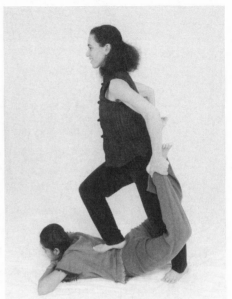

140. Pull Both Legs Up

your right foot on the sacrum and pull the leg up a little. Then lower the leg a little. Repeat with your foot on the lumbar back. The second time, pull the leg up a little higher than you did the first time. Lower the leg a little. Move your foot higher up the lumbar back and repeat. This pull should be the highest. Lower the leg a little. Then go back in the reverse order. The full pattern is 1-2-3-2-1. Repeat the technique on the opposite side.

140. Pull Both Legs Up

This technique extends the lower regions of the spine, making it more flexible, and increases the mobility of the hip joints. It also stretches the quadriceps and iliopsoas muscles. Raising the legs increases the circulation of blood back toward the heart.

Stand behind the recipient's feet. Pick up the ankles and, holding the legs up, walk between the legs almost up to the groin. Raise the left leg a little and slide your left foot under the thigh. Place your right foot on the sacrum and pull the legs up and forward. As you pull up, bend your arms at the elbows and lean forward. Lower the legs a little. Repeat with the ball of your foot on the spine in the lumbar region. Then lower the legs a little. Move your foot up the spine to the thoracic (chest) region and repeat. Then repeat the sequence in the reverse order. The whole pattern is 1-2-3-2-1.

141. Sit between the Recipient's Legs (Optional)

These techniques relax the muscles of the back, buttocks, and legs; mobilize the hip and pelvis; and are good for sciatica.

A. Roll Your Forearm on the Back

With your left hand, hold the recipient's left ankle and pick up the left leg. Place your right hand on the mat to support yourself and then slide your right leg under the leg as near to the groin as possible. Sit with your legs bent to the side and back, Thai style. (See Chapter 7.) Place the leg over your thighs, which will raise the pelvis on that side. Place your right forearm on the left lumbar waist and your left hand on the buttock or thigh. Roll your forearm on the left side of the lumbar (lower) back.

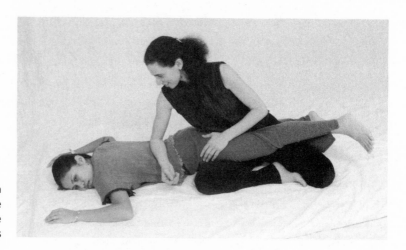

141A. Roll Your Forearm on the Back While Sitting Between the Recipient's Legs

B. Press Your Elbow on the Buttock

Place your right elbow on the recipient's left buttock. Press in with your elbow. Move your elbow to another place on the buttock and lean in again. In

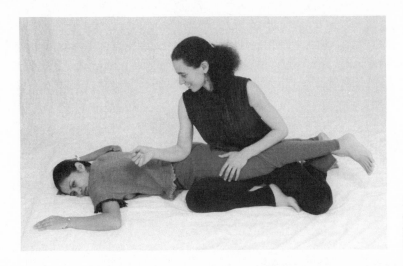

141B. Press Your Elbow on the Buttocks while Sitting Between the Recipient's Legs

this way, elbow press on the buttock. You can also work along the left side of the sacrum and just below the left ischial tuberosity (the "sit bone").

C. Walk Your Elbows on the Leg

Interlace your fingers. Place your right elbow on the recipient's leg below the buttock and your left elbow by the ankle. Walk your elbows in toward each other and then out. Repeat this a few times.

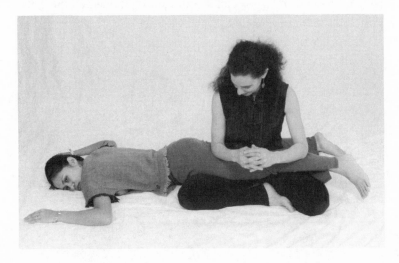

141C. Walk Your Elbows on the Leg while Sitting Between the Recipient's Legs

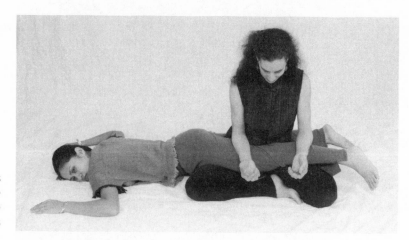

141D. Roll Your Forearms
on the Leg While
Sitting Between the
Recipient's Legs

D. Roll Your Forearms on the Leg

Place your forearms on the recipient's thigh and calf. Then roll them away from each other. Repeat this several times.

E. Chop Your Hands on the Back and Legs

Put your palms together with your thumbs interlaced and your fingers spread open. Chop up and down the back, buttocks, and legs.

Note: To get out of this position, hold the recipient's left ankle with your left hand. Bend the leg and, with your right hand on the mat for support, slide out of the position.

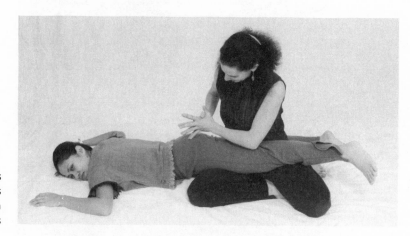

141E. Chop Your Hands
on the Back and Legs
While Sitting Between
the Recipient's Legs

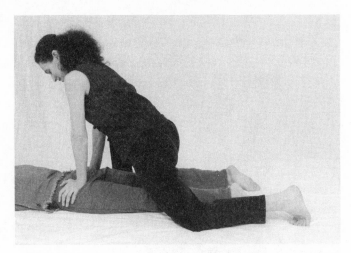

142. Palm Press on the Buttocks

When you have completed all of the steps of technique 141 on one side of the recipient's body, repeat them on the other side.

142. Palm Press on the Buttocks (Optional)

This technique relaxes the buttocks.

Come to a half-lunge position over the recipient's body. Place your hands on the buttocks and palm press them simultaneously or one after the other.

143. Elbow Press on the Buttock (Optional)

This technique relaxes the buttocks.

Kneel or sit Thai style by the right side of the recipient's buttocks and place your left elbow on the left buttock. Lean in. Repeat with your elbow at different places on the buttock. Repeat on the other side.

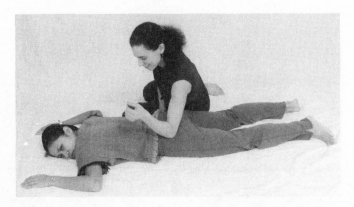

143. Elbow Press on the Buttock

144. Knee Press on the Side of the Buttock (Optional)

This technique relaxes the buttock, specifically the gluteus medius muscle.

Kneel facing the recipient's hips. Place one of your knees on the left side of the buttocks. Place your hands on the right side of the buttocks. Press in with your knee as you simultaneously pull your hands toward you. Move your knee to another place on the side of the buttocks and repeat. Then repeat on the other side.

145. Knee Press on the Buttocks (Optional)

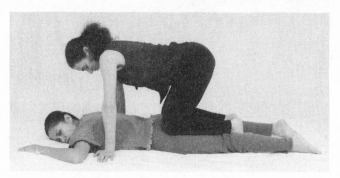

145. Knee Press on the Buttocks

This technique relaxes the buttocks.

Place both of your knees on the recipient's buttocks with your feet between the legs and your hands on the mat. Lean in. Move your knees to another place on the buttocks and repeat. To increase the pressure, you can raise your feet off of the mat so that all of your weight is on your knees.

146. Palm Circle on the Buttocks (Optional)

This technique relaxes the buttocks.

Straddle the recipient in a half-kneeling, half-lunging position. Place your palms on the sides of the buttocks and circle.

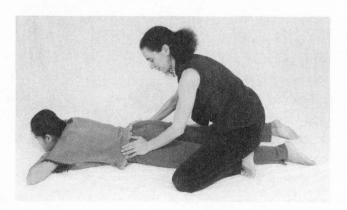

146. Palm Circle on
the Buttocks

147. Palpate the Spine (Optional)

This technique acquaints you with the spine's condition.

Kneel to the side of the recipient. Place your palm on the back, with your middle finger on the spine. Slide your hand down the back, feeling for the spine's condition, noticing whether it is straight or curved.

148. Palm Press on the Back

This technique mobilizes the spine and relaxes the back, specifically the erector spinae, latissimus dorsi, trapezius, rhomboid, and quadratus lumborum muscles. It is a good way to feel the condition of the back. Notice if the rib cage is symmetrical or if one side is higher than the other. Notice where the back is tight and where it is relaxed.

Come to a half-lunge position over the recipient's body. Place your hands in the butterfly position on the lumbar (lower) back, with the heels of your hands on either side of the spine. Palm press with both of your hands simultaneously up and down the back. Repeat a few times.

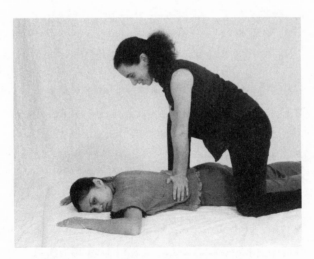

148. Palm Press on the Back

149. Palm Press on the Back with Lower Legs
Interlocked (Optional)

This technique relaxes the back muscles and mobilizes the spine.

Bend the recipient's legs. Stand on the thighs just above the knees and

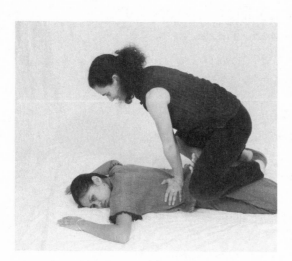

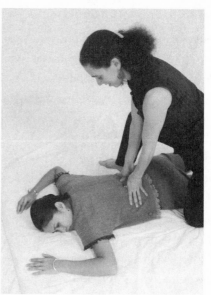

149. Palm Press on the Back with Lower Legs Interlocked

150. Thumb Press on the Back Line

interlock his or her lower legs with your legs. Bend your knees and come to a squatting position. Palm press up and down the back as you lean forward.

150. Thumb Press on the Back Line

This technique relaxes the back muscles, stimulates the flow of energy along the Back Line, and stimulates the paraspinal nerves.

Come to a half-lunge position over the recipient's body. Thumb press up and down the back next to the spine with both of your thumbs simultaneously.

151. Thumb Roll over the Erector Spinae Muscles (Optional)

This technique relaxes the erector spinae muscles.

Kneel at the side of the recipient. Place your thumbs on the outer side of the erector spinae muscles closest to you and press down a little, then roll over the muscles. Repeat a few times. Then place your thumbs on the other side of the back on the inner side of the erector spinae muscles and roll over them. Repeat a few times.

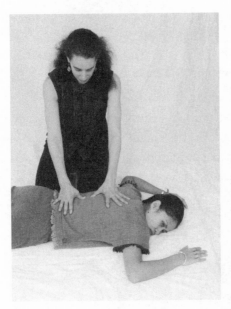

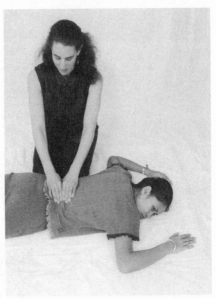

151. Thumb Roll over the Erector Spinae Muscles

152. Squeeze the Lower Back

Then move to the other side of the recipient and repeat from the other side.

152. Squeeze the Lower Back (Optional)

This technique relaxes the lower back.

Kneel at the side of the recipient facing the waist. Place your hands on the lower back and squeeze a few times.

153. Forearm on the Back (Optional)

This technique relaxes the back.

Sit Thai style by the left side of the recipient's back. Place your right forearm on the right side of the back with your hand facing you. Lean on the back. Then move your forearm to another place on the back and lean again. Repeat as you go up the back. When you come to the shoulder blades, lean in between them with your elbow. Then go down the back in the reverse.

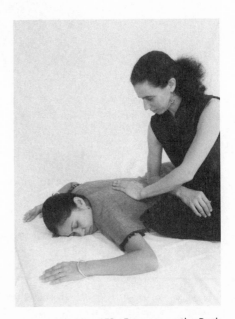

153. Forearm on the Back

Repeat technique 153 on the opposite side, with your hand facing away from you.

154. Knee Press on the Back (Optional)

This technique relaxes the back.

Place your hands on the recipient's upper back and buttock. Place one of your knees on the back and knee press with it up and down the back. Then, if the back is strong enough, place your other knee on the back and walk the two knees alternately.

Repeat on the opposite side.

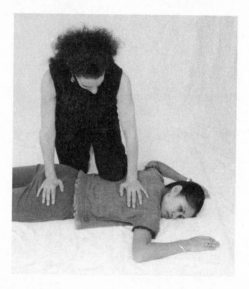

154. Knee Press
on the Back

155. Walk on the Body (Optional)

These techniques relax the back, buttocks, and thighs, and mobilize the spine.

A. On the Thighs

Stand on the recipient's thighs, facing the head, and walk on them.

B. On the Buttocks

Walk on the recipient's buttocks.

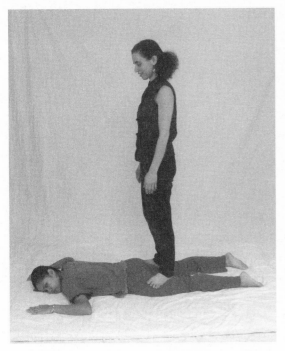

155A. Walk on the Thighs

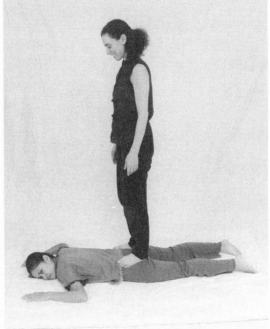

155B. Walk on the Buttocks

C. On the Back

Stand with one foot on the recipient's buttock. Place your other foot on the back and press on different places on the back. Change the position of your feet and walk on the back with your other foot.

Note: To keep your balance when doing foot walking, it helps to put a chair next to the recipient and to hold on to the back edge of the chair.

156. Sit on the Recipient's Feet (Optional)

Techniques A, B, and C relax the back muscles and stimulate energy flow in the body. Technique D expands the chest, which in turn improves the

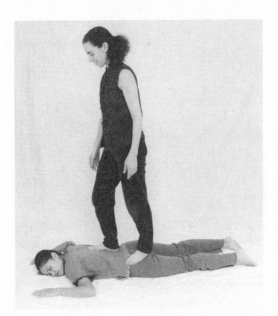

155C. Walk on the Back

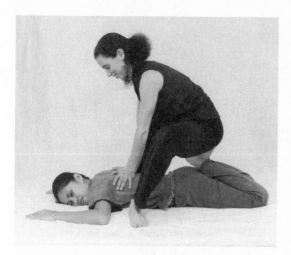

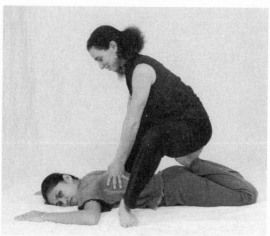

156A. Palm Press on the Back while Sitting on the Recipient's Feet

156B. Thumb Press on the Back while Sitting on the Recipient's Feet

breathing, and also mobilizes the spine and shoulder complex, and stretches the pectoralis major and abdominal muscles.

A. Palm Press on the Back

Bend the recipient's legs at the knees and bring the feet toward the buttocks. Straddle the recipient's body and sit on the feet with your feet by the side of the chest. Press up and down the back with your palms on either side of the back.

B. Thumb Press on the Back

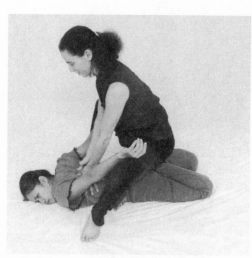

Thumb press up and down the back with your thumbs in the grooves on either side of the spine.

C. Thumb Press with the Arms Raised

Lift the recipient's arms up and place the wrists on your thighs. Repeat the thumb presses up and down the back in the grooves by the sides of the spine.

156C. Thumb Press with the Arms Raised

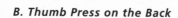

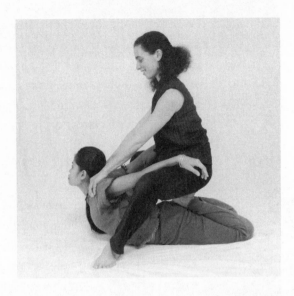

156D. Pull the Chest Up

D. Pull the Chest Up

Place your hands below the recipient's shoulders. As the recipient inhales, pull the shoulders back toward you, lifting the chest. As the recipient exhales, lower the shoulders, returning him or her to the mat. Repeat two more times. Return the arms to the mat and get off the recipient's feet. Place the feet on the mat.

157. Recipient's Arm Up on Your Leg

A. Thumb Press on the Back

Half lunge over the recipient in whichever direction his or her face is turned: For example, if the recipient's face is turned to the left, step over the body with your left leg. Lift the left arm up and place it on your left thigh. Place your thumbs on the Back Line, with your thumbs facing each other. Swivel the fingers of your

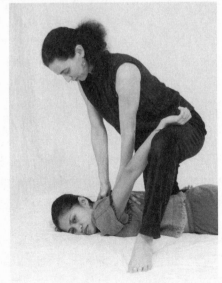

157A. Thumb Press on the Back

right hand clockwise so that they aren't in the recipient's face but rather on the back. The swiveled hand position is used only when you are working the upper back to prevent your fingers from going in the face. Thumb press down and up the back with both of your thumbs simultaneously. Repeat in areas where you find stiffness. As you thumb press, lean forward. This will move the recipient's arm a little toward his or her head.

B. Pull the Shoulder Back while Palm Pressing on the Lower Back

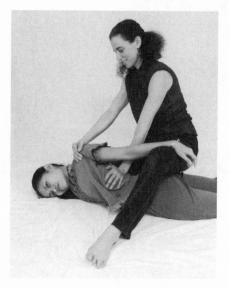

157B. Pull the Shoulder Back while Palm Pressing on the Lower Back

This technique rotates the spine, mobilizes the shoulder complex, opens up the chest, and relaxes the back muscles.

With your right hand, hold the recipient's left shoulder. Place your left hand below the shoulder blade with your fingers pointing out. Pull the shoulder up and back toward you as you simultaneously press on the thoracic back (chest-level area) with your other hand. The pressure of your hands pulling and pushing should be equal when doing these two different movements. Lower the shoulder a little. Move your left hand down the back a little. Pull the recipient's shoulder up and back toward you again, a little more than you did the first time. Simultaneously press on the back. Repeat the above one more time with your left hand now on the lumbar (lower) back. This pull should be the strongest. Then repeat the steps in the reverse order. The whole pattern is 1-2-3-2-1.

Repeat the entire technique on the opposite side.

158. Cobra Pose

These techniques extend the upper region of the spine and the pelvis, bringing more suppleness to the spine. They also expand the chest cavity, thus improving the health of the lungs; mobilize the shoulder complex; and elongate the tissues of the front of the trunk.

A. Palm Press on the Back and Arms

Place both of the recipient's arms by his or her sides. Kneel on the person's thighs just below the buttocks. Have your feet together between the recipi-

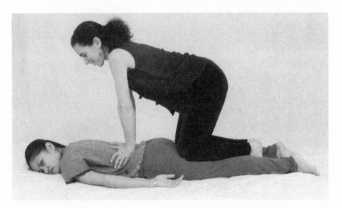

158A. Palm Press the Back and Arms

ent's legs. Palm press up the back and then palm press walk down, up, and down the arms, ending at the wrists.

B. Cobra: Pull the Arms Back while Lifting the Chest Up

Hold the recipient's hands or forearms. Lean back, pulling the arms toward you as you raise the chest up. Do not press with your knees on the thighs—just rest them there lightly. Then relax the pull, lowering the recipient down. Move your knees back a little bit. Then lean back again, pulling the arms toward you a little more than you did the first time. Relax the pull again, lowering the back to the mat. Repeat one more time, with your knees just a little bit further down the thighs. This time, the recipient should reach the maximum extension that is comfortable for him or her—do not go beyond this.

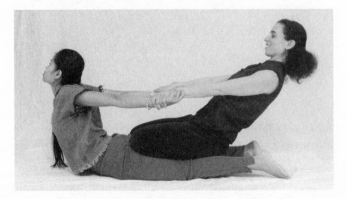

158B. Cobra: Pull the Arms Back While Lifting the Chest Up

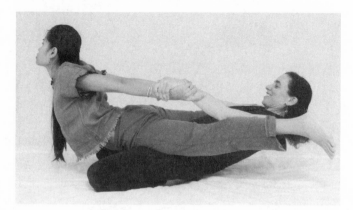

158C. Cobra Variation 1: Legs Behind the Back

C. Cobra: Variation 1: Legs Behind the Back

Pick up the recipient's legs and slide your knees under them. Hold the hands or forearms and then pull them back toward you as you lean back. Lower them to the mat. Repeat two more times.

158D. Cobra Variation 2: Legs Interlocked Behind the Back

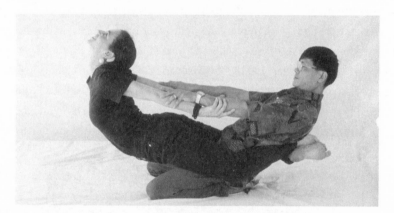

D. Cobra Variation 2: Legs Interlocked Behind the Back

Have the recipient interlock his or her ankles behind your back. Pull the recipient back. As you pull back, lean against the legs. Lower the recipient to the mat. Repeat two more times.

Note: The recipient should grip his or her buttocks during this movement if he or she has any lower back disk problems.

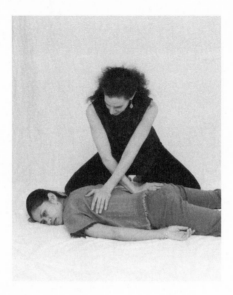

159. Cross Stretch the Back

159. Cross Stretch the Back (Optional)

This technique creates more space between the vertebrae.

Place one of your hands on the recipient's pelvis and your other hand on the back on the opposite side. Diagonally stretch the back. Move your hands further apart and repeat. Do this one more time. Then change the position of your hands so that they are on opposite sides of the back and repeat the three diagonal stretches.

160. Child Pose (Optional)

This technique creates more space between the vertebrae and is a good counterpose for the previous positions, which extended the spine.

Have the recipient come to the position known as the child pose in yoga, which is kneeling with the head down. Kneel behind the recipient and press down on the pelvis with your hands.

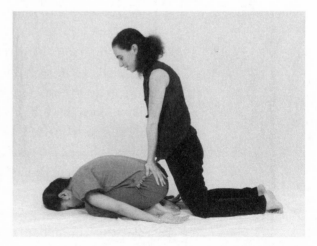

160. Child Pose

CHAPTER

12

THE TRADITIONAL SEQUENCE: THE INVERTED POSITION

The reason why love and compassion bring the greatest happiness is simply that our nature cherishes them above all else. The need for love lies at the very foundation of our human existence. It results from the profound interdependence we all share with one another.

—His Holiness The Dalai Lama

The basic inverted position is on the back with the legs up.

This position is a lot of fun, as the recipient is put into all sorts of interesting positions. This part of the treatment really feels like a dance. As the legs are above the level of the head in most of the exercises, this section is known as the inverted section, even though in many cases the person is not fully inverted. Since the postures are not held for long periods of time as they are in yoga, the benefits and risks are not as strong. However, it is good to know that inversion revitalizes the whole system, improves circulation, stimulates the functioning of the internal organs, and relieves strain on the legs.

Note: The inverted position is contraindicated for people who have high blood pressure or heart disease, or who are menstruating.

161. Assisted Shoulder Stand

This technique aids digestion, massages the back, mobilizes the spine, and increases the flow of blood to the heart and brain. It is good for people with low blood pressure.

Have the recipient lie on his or her back. Pick up both of the legs and hold both ankles with one of your hands. Stand with your left leg behind the recipient and your right leg by his or her side. Have the recipient put his or her hands on the thighs, just above the knees. Tell the recipient to keep his or her arms locked as you roll them up. Rock the recipient forward and back three times. Each succeeding rock should be a little bigger than the previous one.

Note: Do not use this technique on a person who has high blood pressure, heart disease, or cervical damage, or who is menstruating.

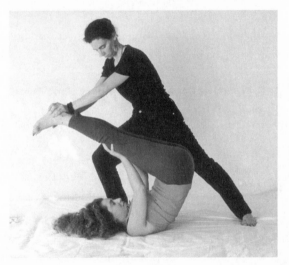

161. Assisted Shoulder Stand

162. Assisted Plow (Optional)

This technique mobilizes the spine and gives it an extra supply of blood due to the forward bend. The abdominal organs are compressed, which massages and rejuvenates them. The gastrocnemius (calf), hamstring, and back muscles are stretched.

Have the recipient place his or her arms on the mat. With your right

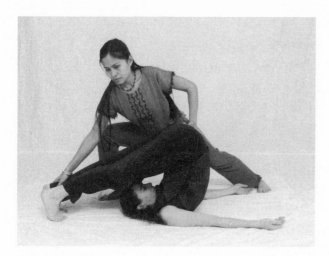

162. Assisted Plow

hand, hold the ankles. Bring the legs overhead down toward the mat. Place your left hand on the person's sacrum.

163. Forward Rock with One Leg Bent

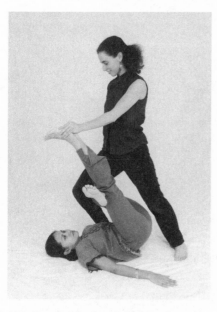

163. Forward Rock with One Leg Bent

This technique mobilizes the spine and the hip joint of the bent leg.

Hold the recipient's legs up. Bring your right knee behind the left knee to bend the leg. Place the left ankle on the front of the right thigh. Step over the bent leg with your right leg. Hold the right heel with your left hand and rock the leg forward at a slight angle toward the left shoulder. When pushing the leg forward, first straighten your arm and then lean forward. Also, as you rock forward, raise your right heel up and bend your leg more so as to give the bent leg more room to move forward. Bring the recipient back. Move your right foot forward a little. Rock the recipient forward again. Repeat the procedure one more time. The third rock should be the biggest. At the end of the third rock forward, intensify the stretch by placing your left hand on the recipient's right buttock and your right hand on the right heel and then pushing your hands in opposite directions. When you do the stretch, the extended leg should be at a slight angle toward the shoulder.

164. One Leg Bent and Held in Place (Optional)

This technique mobilizes the hip joint of the bent leg.

Prepare for this as you did for technique 163. Try to move the extended leg forward, but this time do not bend your right leg. Your right leg should act like a brace against the bent leg, which will not be able to move forward now. Repeat a few times.

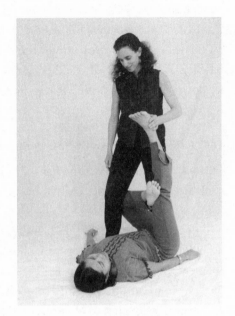

164. One Leg Bent and Held in Place

165. Forearm Press on the Sole

This technique stretches the Achilles tendon and the hamstring and calf muscles.

Your leg position here is similar to the one in technique 164. Bring your right leg back as much as possible, locking the recipient's bent leg in place. Place the right extended leg at the middle of your abdomen, and keep it in place from behind with your left leg. Place your right forearm on the recipient's sole and hold the foot from underneath with your left hand. Your right elbow should not extend beyond the inner side of the foot. Bring your chest for-

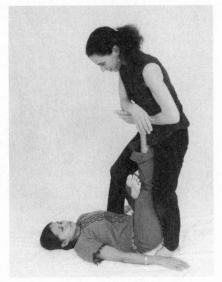

165. Forearm Press on the Sole

ward as you lean on the foot. Press with your forearm on various places on the sole of the foot. Each time you press, make sure to lean forward from your chest.

Note: If the recipient's legs are very long and you have trouble leaning on the sole, go up on your tiptoes. If this does not work, do not lock the bent leg in place. Instead, stand behind the two legs and bring the extended leg down toward you until it is at a comfortable height for you to sole press on. Then work on it.

166. Forward Rock with Your Knee on the Bent Leg

This technique mobilizes the hip joints and softens the adjoining tissues, stretches the back of the straight leg, and works on the attachments of the hamstrings on the bent leg.

Step behind the recipient's bent leg. Rest the recipient's extended right leg on your left arm—not on your shoulder. Place your right hand on the recipient's left knee and your left hand on the recipient's left ankle. Angle the knee in toward the sternum (breastbone) a little. Place your right knee on the back of the left thigh just above the "sit bone," with your right foot out to the side, and have your left foot on the mat behind the recipient. Do not apply much pressure through your right knee—it is just there for support. Rock the recipient forward as you simultaneously move your shoulder

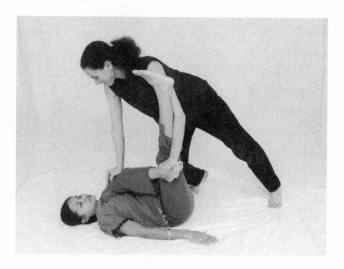

166. Forward Rock with Your Knee on the Bent Leg

forward to increase the stretch on the straight leg. Bring the recipient back toward you and then move your knee a little higher up on the back of the thigh. Rock the recipient forward again as you move your shoulder forward. Bring the recipient back again. Place your knee where it was originally and repeat the procedure. The whole pattern is 1-2-1.

When you have completed techniques 163 through 166 on one side of the recipient's body, repeat them on the other side.

167. Forearm Press on the Soles (Optional)

This technique stretches the Achilles tendon and the calf and hamstring muscles.

Position the recipient with both legs up in the air. Stand behind the recipient. With your forearms, lean on the soles of the feet, especially on the balls of the feet.

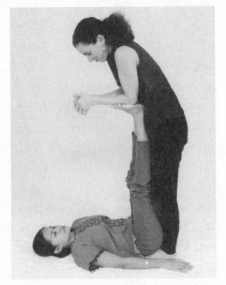

167. Forearm Press on the Soles

168. Hamstring Stretch with Bent Legs

This technique stretches the hamstring muscles.

With both of the recipient's legs up and bent, hold the heels. Place your knees on the backs of the thighs just above the "sit bones." Your feet should be spread apart. Stretch the recipient's legs forward. Bring the legs back a little to release the stretch. Then move your knees up the thighs without changing the position of your feet and stretch the legs for-

168. Hamstring Stretch with Bent Legs

ward again. Bring the legs back again and move your knees still further up the thighs without changing the position of your feet. Stretch the legs forward once more. Then repeat the steps in the reverse order, moving your knees down to just above the "sit bones." The whole pattern is 1-2-3-2-1.

169. Hamstring Stretch with Straight Legs (Optional)

This technique stretches the hamstring muscles.

Stand behind the recipient's straight legs, which should be up in the air. Hold the heels. Place your knees on the recipient's buttocks just above the "sit bones." Push the legs forward. Release the forward stretch a little and move your knees slightly up on the backs of the thighs. Push the legs forward again. Repeat one more time with your knees back at the original position. The pattern is 1-2-1.

170. The Bridge

This technique strengthens the back, gives the spine a backward stretch, gives the head and neck a vascular flush, and stretches the quadriceps and rectus abdominis (stomach) muscles.

Bend the recipient's legs at the knees and bring the legs toward the

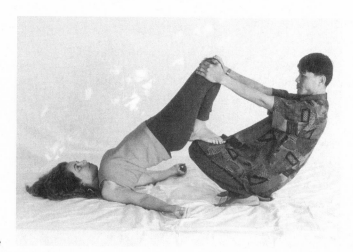

170. The Bridge

chest. Stand behind the feet. Put your knees together and your feet out, forming a triangle. Place the feet on your knees. Hold the knees with one hand on each knee and then slowly squat down. As you go down, the insteps will roll over your knees and the back and pelvis will rise up off of the floor. Hold the posture for a few seconds. Slowly stand up and then repeat two more times.

171. Bound Angle

These techniques open up the hip joints.

A. Feet Toward the Nose

Hold the recipient's ankles and pick up the legs. Step through the legs next to the armpits. Bring the feet together in front of you. As the recipient exhales, push the feet down toward the nose with your arms straight. Relax the pressure a little. Repeat two more times.

B. Feet Overhead

As the recipient exhales, push the feet down over the head. Relax the pressure a little. Repeat two more times.

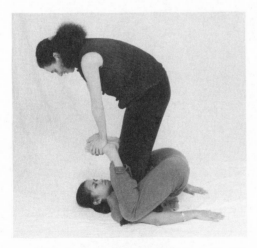
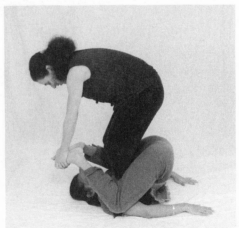

171A. Feet Toward the Nose in Bound Angle   171B. Feet Overhead in Bound Angle

172. Sit-ups over Your Knees (Optional)

This technique stretches the back and spine, strengthens the abdominal tissues, and stimulates the flexor muscles of the trunk.

A. Legs Up

Have the recipient lie on his or her back with legs overhead in the plow position. Squat behind the recipient and balance on the balls of your feet. Place your knees on the lumbar (lower) back. Hold the hips and then bring the legs up overhead.

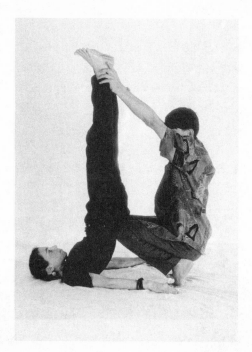

172A. Legs Up

B. Assisted Bridge

Open the recipient's legs and bring them down toward you over your thighs and then place the feet on the mat. Hold the knees and lie down.

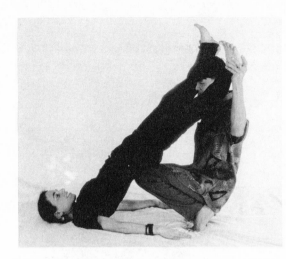

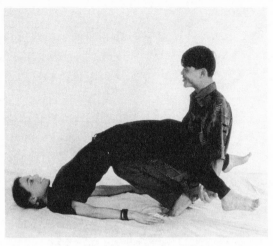

172B. Assisted Bridge

C. Sit-ups

Have the recipient interlace his or her hands behind the neck. Hold the knees firmly and have the recipient sit up. Repeat several times.

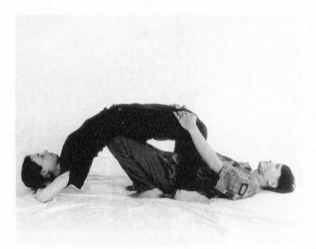

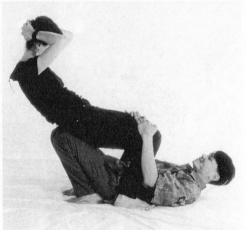

172C. Sit-ups

D. Closure

On the last round, as the recipient goes down to the mat, sit up while holding the legs. Push the feet toward the chest as you quickly stand up. Bring the bent legs to the chest.

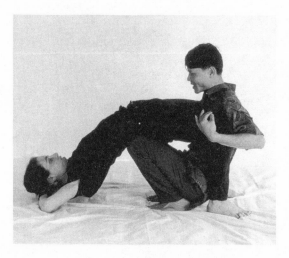 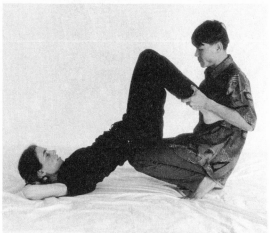

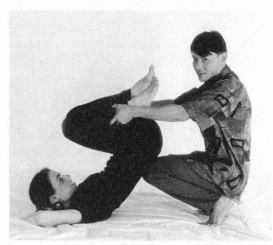 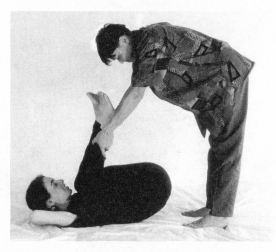

172D. Closure

173. Both Feet Behind Your Knees (Optional)

These techniques relax the quadriceps muscles. For the practitioner, it mobilizes the spine, stretches the anterior tissues of the trunk, opens and expands the chest, and strengthens the abdominal muscles.

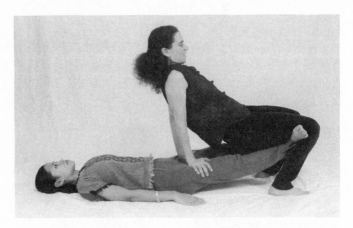

173A. Walk Hands on the Thighs

A. Walk Hands on the Thighs

Stand at the recipient's feet and face away. Pick up the legs and place the feet behind your knees. Bend your legs to hold the feet in place behind your knees. Place your hands behind you on the thighs and bend backward as you walk your hands up and down the thighs.

B. Back Arch Holding Recipient's Thighs

Place your hands at about the middle of the recipient's thighs. Arch your back up and drop your head back. When you have finished, come back to a standing position in preparation for the next technique.

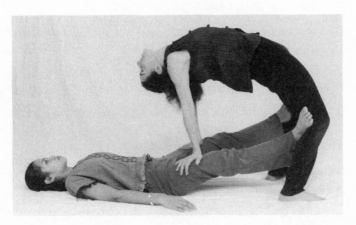

173B. Back Arch Holding Recipient's Thighs

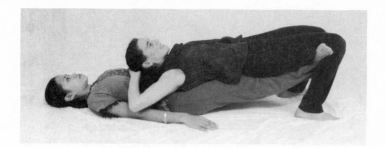

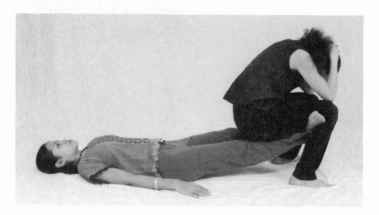

173C. Sit-ups on the
Recipient's Legs

C. Sit-ups on the Recipient's Legs

Lie down on the recipient's legs. Interlace your fingers and place your hands behind your head. Sit up on the legs. Repeat several times.

174. Pull-up with Legs Straight (Optional)

This technique mobilizes the hip joint and shoulder complex and stretches the hamstring muscles.

Lift the recipient's legs and put them on your legs and/or chest, depending on how far the legs reach. Hold the wrists and pull the recipient up. Then lower the recipient to the mat. Repeat two more times.

175. Pull-up with Legs Crossed

This technique mobilizes the hip and knee joints and the shoulder complex. It also acts as a connecting move to the sitting position.

Bend both of the recipient's legs and cross them at the ankles. Stand in

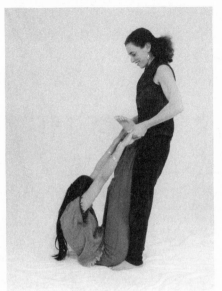 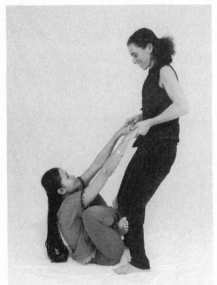

174. Pull-up with Legs Straight   175. Pull-up with Legs Crossed

front of the recipient and place his or her ankles below your knees. Have your knees together and your feet apart. Hold the recipient's hands. Pull the recipient up to you, then lower him or her. Repeat two more times. The third time, after pulling the recipient up, walk back a few steps so that the recipient ends up in a sitting position.

CHAPTER

13

THE TRADITIONAL
SEQUENCE: THE
SEATED POSITION

*Those engaged in the practice of compassion feel much happier
internally—more calm, more peaceful—and other people
reciprocate that feeling.* —His Holiness The Dalai Lama

The basic seated position is with the ankles crossed and the back
straight. The hands should be relaxed at the sides or in the lap.

The seated position is the last position used in Thai massage. In the
West, where people live very sedentary lives and often sit for long hours in
front of computers, tension tends to accumulate in the shoulders and neck.
Since the shoulders are completely accessible in the seated position, this position is very good for shoulder and neck work. Another benefit of ending
the session with the seated position is that it leaves the recipient ready for
meditation. Make sure the recipient sits with his or her spine straight.

176. Lean on the Shoulders

This technique facilitates energy flow through the shoulders and neck
and relaxes the muscles there, specifically the upper trapezius and levator
scapula muscles.

Have the recipient bend his or her head forward a little. Stand at some

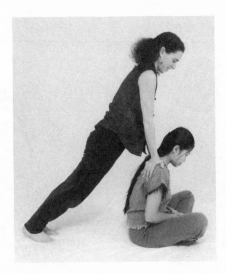

176. Lean on the
Shoulders

distance behind the person. Place your hands on the recipient's shoulders, just beside the neck, with your fingers facing you. Lean forward on the shoulders. Your arms should be straight. Move your hands out a little on the shoulders and lean again. Move your hands still further out and lean again. Then repeat this sequence in the reverse order. The full pattern is 1-2-3-2-1.

Note: Your hands should always be on the shoulder muscles, not on the bones there, so do not go too far out on the shoulders. In this exercise, feel for the condition of these muscles.

177. Thumb Press along the Spine

This technique relaxes the upper back, specifically the upper trapezius and erector spinae muscles, stimulates acupressure points along the sides of the spine, and activates nerve pathways.

Stand a little way behind the recipient. Place your hands on the back with your thumbs facing up on either side of the spine by the shoulders. Lean forward. Move your thumbs down the spine a little way and lean forward again. Reverse the direction of your thumbs so that your thumbs now face down. Lean forward. Move your thumbs down a little more and lean forward again. Move your thumbs still further down, near the lower border of the shoulder blade, and lean forward again. Then reverse the procedure

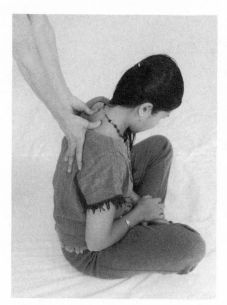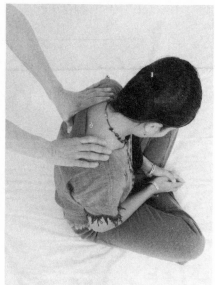

177. Thumb Press along the Spine

going back up in the same way that you came down. The whole pattern is 1-2-3-4-5-4-3-2-1.

178. Arm Overhead and Pulled Back

This technique mobilizes the shoulder complex and the adjoining tissues and helps to relax the shoulder and expand the chest.

Kneel behind the recipient, facing sideward to the right, with your right knee down on the mat and your left knee squatting. This acts as a support for the back. Bring the recipient's left arm up overhead and bend it at the elbow. Hold the recipient's left hand with your left hand, with palm facing palm. Also hold the hand with your right hand. Place your left elbow on the recipient's left shoulder and then pull the arm toward you at about a forty-five-degree angle. Then bring the arm back to its starting position. Move your elbow down the back a little, between the shoulder blade and spine, and pull the arm toward you again. Let the arm back again. Move your elbow a little further down the back and repeat the movement again. Then repeat the sequence in the reverse order. The full pattern is 1-2-3-2-1.

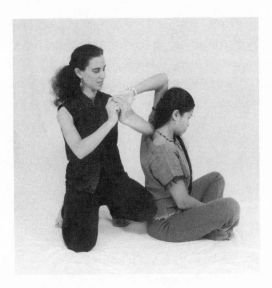

178. Arm Overhead and Pulled Back

Note: This technique can also be done while kneeling behind the recipient with both knees open as you face the recipient's back.

179. Pull the Arm Back

This technique stretches the side of the body, opens the chest, extends the spine, mobilizes the shoulder joint, and stretches the triceps muscle.

A. Pull the Arm

Stand sideways behind the recipient, with your right leg by the recipient's spine and your left leg back and slightly to the side. The recipient's arm is still bent at the elbow. With your right hand, hold the elbow. Place your left hand on the upper arm near the armpit. Pull the arm back with your right hand and supplement the movement with your left hand. As you pull, simultaneously bend your right leg a little, pushing your knee into the recipient's back to extend it. Your knee should be on the same side of the back as the arm that is raised. Then release the pull along with the knee push. Move your left hand up the arm a little and repeat.

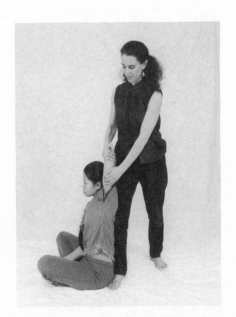

179A. Pull the Arm

Move your left hand still further up the arm toward the elbow and repeat. Then repeat the sequence in the reverse order, moving your left hand back toward the armpit. The full pattern is 1-2-3-2-1.

Note: With this technique, it is your right hand that does most of the work; your left hand just adds to the pulling movement.

B. Tapotement

With your left hand in a loose fist, hit up and down on the upper arm.

180. Rotate the Arm and Cross Stretch (Optional)

These techniques improve shoulder flexibility and facilitate increased circulation to the shoulder complex.

A. Rotate the Arm

Kneel behind the recipient. Hold the recipient's left wrist with your left hand and place your right hand on the shoulder. Rotate the arm counterclockwise a few times. As you bring the arm back, simultaneously push the shoulder forward.

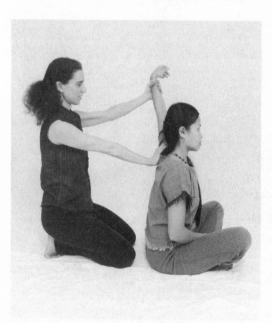

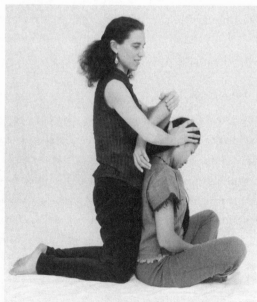

180A. Rotate the Arm   180B. Cross Stretch

B. Cross Stretch

Bring the recipient's arm behind the head. Place your left hand on the elbow and your right hand on the right side of the head. Push the arm and head in opposite directions.

181. Thumb Press (Optional)

These techniques mobilize the shoulder blade and soften adjoining tissues.

A. Around the Shoulder Blade

Position yourself behind the recipient, facing his or her back. Kneel on your left knee and squat with your right leg. Bring the left arm behind the back and bend it at the elbow. With your right knee, hold the palm in place. Place your left hand on the shoulder and with your right thumb, press around the left shoulder blade. As you thumb press, simultaneously pull the shoulder toward you.

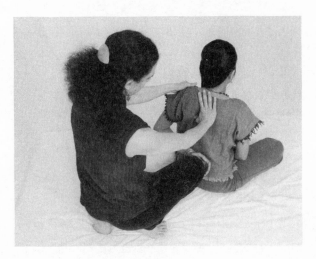

181A. Thumb Press around the Shoulder Blade

B. Thumb Press on the Arm

Hold the recipient's shoulder with your right hand, and with your left hand, thumb press down and up the arm.

When you have completed techniques 178 through 181 on one side of the recipient's body, repeat the entire sequence (or parts of it) on the other side.

182. Stretch Both Arms Overhead (Optional)

This technique increases the mobility of the shoulder complex and opens the chest.

Stand behind the recipient, facing sideways with your right leg by the side of the spine. Hold the wrists and raise the arms overhead. Then pull the arms back toward you.

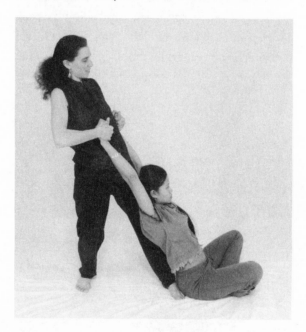

182. Stretch Both Arms Overhead

183. Chest Opener (Optional)

This technique opens up the chest, mobilizes the shoulder joints, and stretches the pectoralis muscles.

A. Pull the Elbows Back

Stand behind the recipient. Have the recipient interlace his or her fingers behind the head. Hold the elbows and pull them back slightly. Release. Repeat a few times.

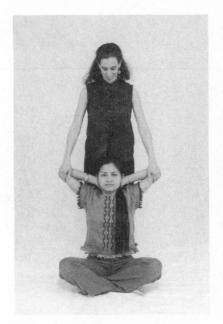

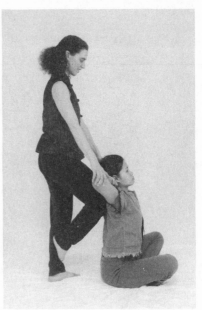

183A. Chest Opener: Pull the Elbows Back

183B. Chest Opener: Knee to Back

B. Knee to Back

To intensify the stretch, place your knee on the recipient's back between the shoulder blades and then pull back. Release. Repeat a few times.

184. Squeeze the Neck with Your Fingers

This technique relaxes the back of the neck.

Half lunge at the right side of the recipient, with your left leg supporting the recipient's back. Place your hands sideways on the neck with your fingers on one side and your thumbs on the other side. Keep your arms outstretched but relaxed. Squeeze the neck between your fingers and thumbs. Squeeze up and down the neck a few times.

When you have completed technique 184 from one side of the recipient's body, repeat it from the other side.

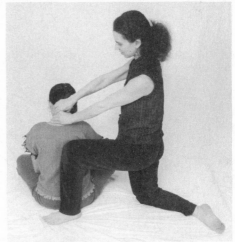

184. Squeeze the Neck with Your Fingers

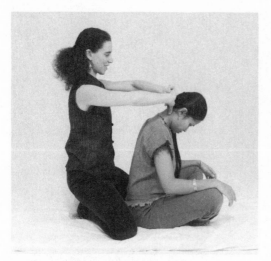

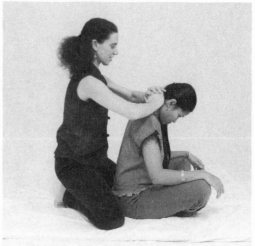

185A. Squeeze the Neck with Your Thumbs

185B. Squeeze the Neck with the Heels of
Your Hands

185. Squeeze the Neck

This technique relaxes the back of the neck.

A. With Your Thumbs

Kneel behind the recipient with your knees spread open. Interlace your fingers and place your thumbs on the recipient's neck. Squeeze up and down the neck with your thumbs.

B. With the Heels of Your Hands

Squeeze the recipient's neck between the heels of your hands, especially using the thenar pads (the fleshy area adjacent to your thumbs).

186. Thumb Press Along the Base of the Skull

This technique can relieve headaches. It relaxes the muscles that attach to the base of the skull, elongates the tissues of the neck, and places traction on the neck.

Kneel on your left knee and half squat with your right leg behind the recipient. Have your squatting knee raised up and use it as a support for your right elbow when you thumb press. Place your left hand on the fore-

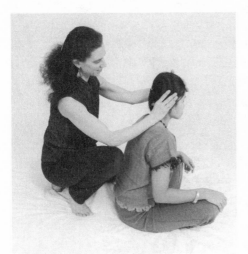 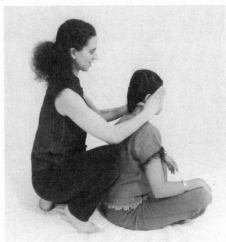

186. Thumb Press Along the Base of the Skull   187. Raise the Head Up

head to stabilize it when you are thumb pressing. Place your right thumb in the hollow at the middle of the base of the skull. Thumb press up as you simultaneously lift the head with your other hand. Move your thumb along the base of the skull to the right and repeat. Move your thumb a little further to the right and repeat. Then repeat the sequence in the reverse order. The whole pattern is 1-2-3-2-1.

When you have completed technique 186 on one side of the recipient's body, repeat it on the other side.

187. Raise the Head Up

This technique places traction on the neck.

Hold the recipient's head between the fingers of both of your hands and your thumbs, which should be under the base of the skull. Lift the head up with your thumbs and fingers. Move your thumbs inward and thumb press up again. Move your thumbs back to where you started and thumb press up again. The whole pattern is 1-2-1.

188. Stretch the Neck to the Side (Optional)

This technique helps to improve flexibility of the cervical spine and softens adjoining tissues.

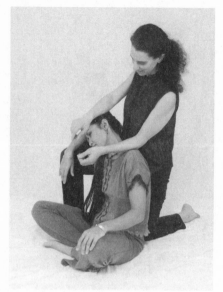
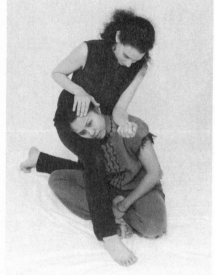

188. Stretch the Neck to the Side

189. Head to the Side on Your Thigh

Come to a half-lunge position with your right knee down on the mat behind the recipient's spine and your left leg on the left side of the recipient. Place the recipient's left arm on your left leg. (This is optional.) Then place your left forearm on the left shoulder just next to the neck. Place your right forearm on the left side of the head. Stretch the shoulder and head away from each other. Move your left forearm a little way down the shoulder and repeat the shoulder and head stretch.

When you have completed technique 188 on one side of the recipient's body, repeat it on the other side.

189. Head to the Side on Your Thigh (Optional)

This technique helps to improve the flexibility of the cervical spine and softens adjoining tissues.

Come to a half-lunge position on the right side of the recipient. Have your left knee down on the mat by the side and your right knee up with that leg in front of the body. Take the head and place it on your right thigh, facing away from you. Hold the head in place with your right hand. With your left elbow, press on the left side of the neck and shoulder.

When you have completed technique 189 on one side of the recipient's body, repeat it on the other side.

190. Massage the Scalp

This technique stimulates the scalp and hair roots, improves blood circulation to the brain, and helps to prevent memory loss. It also helps to prevent insomnia and headaches.

Stand behind the recipient with your left leg supporting the spine and your right leg at the side of the body. Massage the scalp with your fingers.

The Face

Massaging the face helps to prevent wrinkles and premature aging. It increases blood circulation to the face, keeping the skin smooth and supple.

191. Massage the Forehead

This technique relaxes the forehead and can ease headaches.

Rest the heels of your hands on the top of the recipient's head and then finger circle on the forehead from the midline out. Repeat a few times.

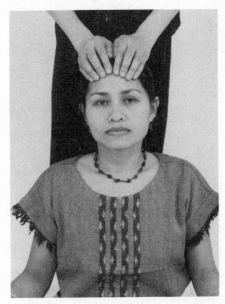

192. Finger Stroke between the Eyebrows

This technique relaxes the area between the eyebrows.

Place your middle fingers between the eyebrows and then finger stroke up between the eyebrows a few times.

191. Massage the Forehead

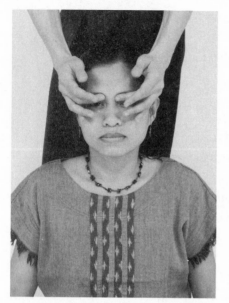

193. Finger Stroke below the Eyebrows

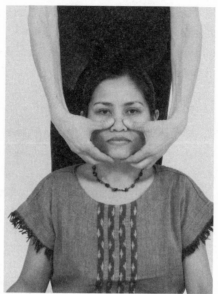

194. Thumb Stroke down the Sides of the Nose

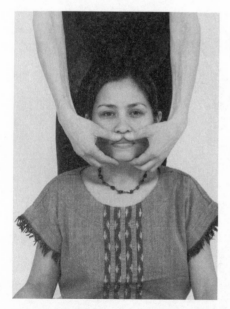

195. Thumb Stroke below the Nose, above the Upper Lip

193. Finger Stroke below the Eyebrows

This technique relaxes the area just under the eyebrows.

Stroke below the recipient's eyebrows with your middle fingers.

194. Thumb Stroke down the Sides of the Nose

This technique relaxes the sides of the nose and can help with nasal congestion.

Place your fingers under the recipient's jaw and your thumbs by the sides of the nose. Thumb stroke down the sides of the nose with one thumb after the other.

195. Thumb Stroke below the Nose, above the Upper Lip

Place your thumbs below the recipient's nose and above the upper lip and thumb stroke outward simultaneously.

196. Massage the Chin and Jaw

This technique relaxes the chin and jaw.

Hold the recipient's chin between your thumbs and fingers, with your fingers under the jaw. With a circular movement of your thumbs, massage in an outward direction from the chin along the jaw. Repeat a few times.

197. Massage the Jaw Muscles

This technique relaxes the masseter (jaw) muscles and is helpful for people who grind their teeth at night.

Place your fingers on the jaw and finger circle there.

198. Twist the Earlobes

This technique relaxes the ears.

Twist the recipient's earlobes at various places.

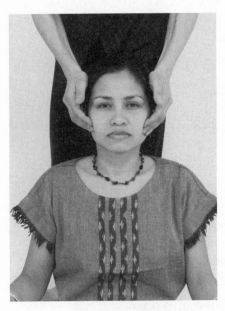
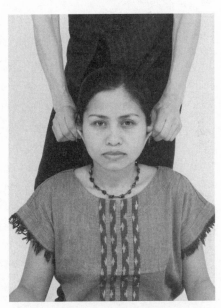

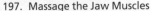

197. Massage the Jaw Muscles   198. Twist the Earlobes

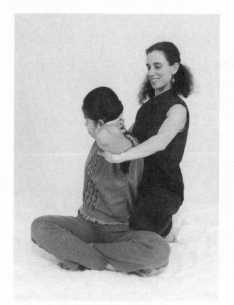

199. Spinal Twist

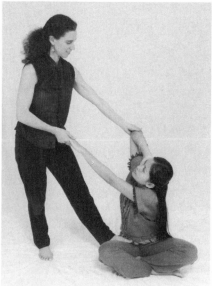

200. With Hand to Ear, Pull the Arm

199. Spinal Twist

This technique helps to mobilize the spine and elongates the adjoining tissues. It also massages the internal organs.

Bring the recipient's hands behind the head and have him or her interlace the fingers. Place your right knee on the mat behind the recipient and your left knee on the recipient's left thigh. Your left knee acts as a brace and should rest lightly. Bring your hands under the recipient's upper arms and then hold the person's forearms near the wrists. Twist the recipient to the right. As you twist the recipient, keep his or her body upright. Then repeat the technique to the other side.

200. With Hand to Ear, Pull the Arm (Optional)

This technique mobilizes the spine and adjoining tissues, opens the chest, and stretches the triceps muscles.

Stand on the right side of the recipient. Have the recipient put his or her right hand on the right ear. Place your left foot on the thigh. With your right hand, hold the left hand and place your left hand on the right elbow. Pull the left arm toward you as you push the right elbow away from you.

201. Knees to the Back

This technique increases spinal extension, opens up the chest, and elongates the tissues in the front of the trunk.

Have the recipient interlace his or her fingers behind the head. Squat behind the recipient, balancing on the balls of your feet. Bring your arms forward under the arms and then slip your hands back through the arms so that you can hold the forearms. Place your knees on the upper thoracic (chest-level) back on either side of the spine. Bring the recipient back toward you. Then move him or her away a little and place your knees further down the back a little and repeat. Repeat with your knees a little further down the back. Then repeat the sequence in the reverse order, going up the back and then down again.

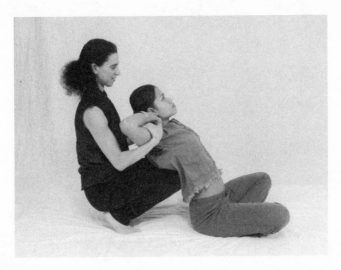

201. Knees to the Back

202. Feet on the Back

This technique loosens up the shoulder blades, increases the flexibility of the spine, opens up the chest, and mobilizes the shoulder complex.

A. On the Spine

Sit behind the recipient. Rotate his or her arms inward and bring the arms behind his or her back and hold the person's hands. Stretch your left leg out and place the outer side of your left foot on the spine. Place your right foot on the sacrum (optional). Then pull the arms toward you against your foot.

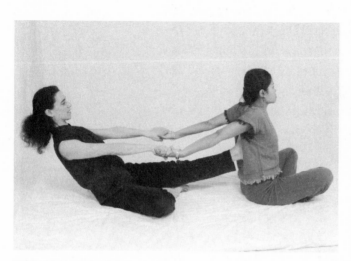

202A. Foot on the Spine

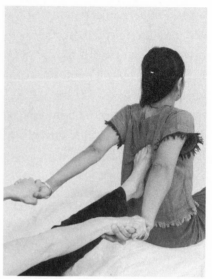

202B. Foot on the Back by the Shoulder Blade

B. By the Shoulder Blade

Place the toes of your left foot by the inner side of the recipient's left shoulder blade and then straighten your leg. Pull the recipient toward you and then relax the pull. Move your left foot to another place by the side of the shoulder blade and repeat. Move your left foot below the shoulder blade and repeat. Then go back up along the side of the shoulder blade in the same way.

Repeat 202A and 202B on the other side of the recipient's body.

C. Both Feet on the Back

Place the soles of your feet on the recipient's thoracic (chest-level) back. Straighten your legs. Pull the arms toward you so that the back is extended by your feet. Relax the pull. Push the arms forward a little. This will make the back go forward so that you can move your feet down the back. Straighten your legs and pull again. Continue in this way down and up the back.

203. Crack the Back (Optional)

This technique mobilizes the spine.

Check to see which one of the recipient's shoulders appears higher than the other. Whichever shoulder is lower, take that arm and cross it in front of the other arm in front of the body. Place your knees on the person's thoracic back and your hands on the elbows. Pull the elbows toward you as you press your knees in and crack the back. Move your knees up to another place on the back and repeat. Continue up the back.

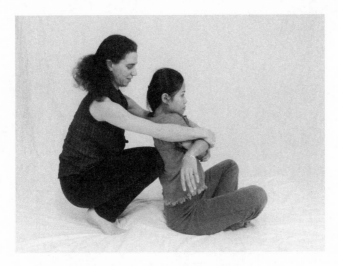

203. Crack the Back

204. Suspended Swing (Optional)

This technique elongates the spine and adjoining tissues, stretches the front tissues of the trunk, and increases blood flow to the head.

A. Standard Version

Have the recipient sit in front of you with his or her fingers interlaced behind the neck. Squat behind the recipient and balance on the balls of your feet. Put your knees on the recipient's lumbar (lower) back. Hold the arms near the armpits. Bring the body back toward you as you roll back onto your back and raise your feet up. The recipient's legs will now drop down. Move the upper body from side to side with your hands.

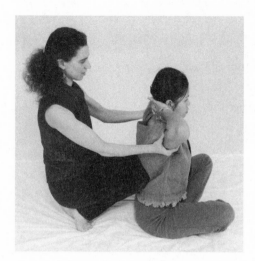

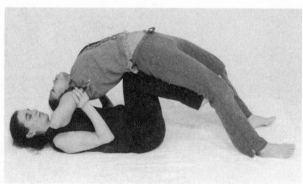

204A. Suspended Swing, Standard Version

B. Variation: With Legs Up

Raise your feet higher than in Step A, so that the recipient's legs are off the mat. The recipient will thus be suspended in space. Swing the recipient from side to side.

205. Back Traction

This technique elongates the spine and adjoining tissues and mobilizes the shoulder complex.

A. Feet on the Sacrum

Sit behind the recipient with your legs extended and the soles of your feet flat on the recipient's sacrum. Place a pillow on your thighs just above your knees. Have the recipient extend his or her legs outward. Have the recipient lie back toward you.

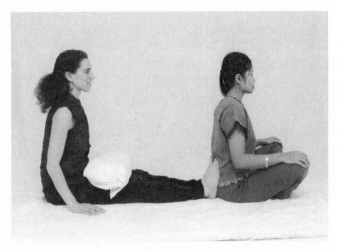

205A. Feet on the Sacrum

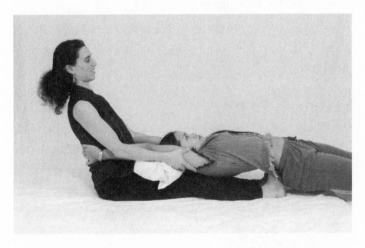

205B. Recipient's Hands on Your Back as You Push Your Feet Forward

B. Recipient's Hands on Your Back as You Push Your Feet Forward

Bring the recipient's arms overhead. Have the recipient hold your back with his or her hands. Hold the arms. Lean back as you simultaneously push the pelvis forward with your feet. Relax your foot push and lean forward a little. Move the recipient's arms down your back a little. Once again, lean back as you push forward with your feet. Repeat with the recipient's hands further down your back. Then repeat the sequence with the recipient's hands going up your back.

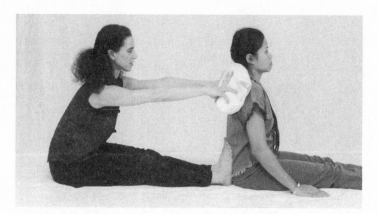

205C. Push the Recipient Up with a Pillow

C. Push the Recipient Up with a Pillow

Bring the recipient's arms back by his or her sides. Put your hands under the pillow. Push the pillow forward quickly. This will bring the recipient back to a seated position.

206. Squeeze the Shoulders

This technique relieves tension in the shoulders and upper back.

Squeeze the recipient's shoulders between your thumbs and fingers. Repeat a few times.

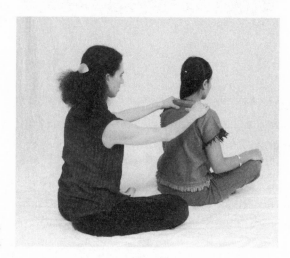

206. Squeeze
the Shoulders

207. Hand Chop on the Back

This technique tones the back muscles and increases blood supply to the area.

Place the fingers of your two hands together with your fingers spread open. Bring your elbows forward. The heels of your palms should be separated. With a loose wrist, chop on the left shoulder and then down and up the left side of the back. Repeat the chopping on the right shoulder and down and up the right side of the back.

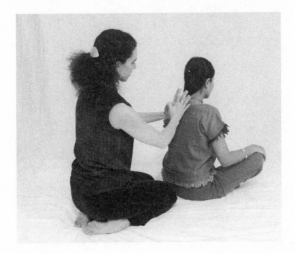

207. Hand Chop on the Back

208. Brush Down the Back and Arms

This technique smooths out the energy in the back and arms and signals the end of the treatment.

Brush down the recipient's back two times with your palms and then brush down the arms.

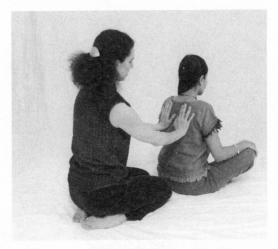

208. Brush Down the Back and Arms

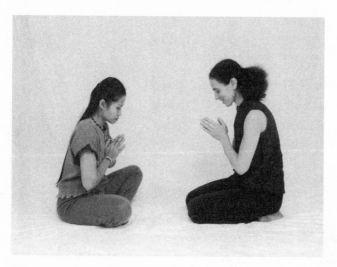

209. Bow in Front of the Recipient

209. Bow in Front of the Recipient

To give closure to the treatment, come around to the front of the recipient, kneel, and bow.

Those engaged in the practice of compassion feel much happier internally—more calm, more peaceful—and other people reciprocate that feeling. —His Holiness The Dalai Lama

APPENDIX:
PICHEST BOONTHUMME,
THAILAND'S MASTER
MASSEUR

Bauw Boonthumme, a traditional Thai doctor and herbalist, and his wife Bauw Jan Boonthumme, who was a cook, gave birth to a baby boy on June 19, 1958. Little did they realize that their son, whom they named Narin, would grow up to become one of Thailand's most sought-after massage therapists and teachers.

They lived in a small village called Hang Dong on a quiet little country lane surrounded by fields, about a half hour from the northern city of Chiangmai. In the garden, Bauw Boonthumme grew mangoes and longans (similar to rambutan). In the surrounding village, artisans worked on ceramics and woodcarving. These, along with the sale of antiques, sustained the village.

When Narin was seven or eight years old, his father began to teach him massage. First he learned how to walk on his father's body so that Bauw could relax before going to bed. Looking back, Narin says this also taught him patience. Bauw continued to teach Narin massage as well as the use of herbs. Narin feels he didn't fully understand his father's lessons until years later, when he was twenty-three or twenty-four years old. At that time, Narin went with his father to Chiangmai.

They went to the Old Medicine Hospital, as Bauw Boonthumme needed to pick up some herbs there. The hospital's director asked Narin if he would like to work at the hospital. Since Narin had no job at the time and had recently married, he gladly accepted the offer. In the beginning, he studied the hospital's massage techniques. Later, in 1983, he was hired as a staff member. He remained at the Old Medicine Hospital until 1990 as a practitioner and teacher.

When Narin was twenty-seven years old, he gave a massage to a monk named Phra Ahjarn Plak Prawit at Wat Ngon in Chiangmai. The monk was very moved by the treatment and felt that Narin truly had the power of massage and really understood spirit. He told Narin he would like to honor him with a new name and chose Pichest, which although it is hard to translate accurately, basically means "special, happy, and good."

In 1990, Pichest decided to start teaching from his home. He was tired of the commute to Chiangmai, which had become increasingly busy due to more and more traffic on the main road. He also longed to have more time to devote to meditation practice.

In the beginning, Pichest taught out of his living room. I was one of his first "home" students. As the living room was very small, Pichest hoped to eventually teach massage at a nearby temple where there would be more space and a religious atmosphere. One day, however, he suddenly had the inspiration that he could build the school on his own land. Within days of having this idea, he began building. A few months later, the structure was complete, and classes began there in 1992.

The school is a long rectangular building made of two rooms. At one end is a classroom with Pichest's shrine area and at the other end is a large shrine room for Pichest's wife. Pichest's dream of having his school in a temple atmosphere had come true.

Whenever a new course begins, all the students and Pichest assemble in front of Pichest's shrine area. Each student makes the traditional offering of white lotus buds, incense, candles, fruit, and money. Pichest then blesses each student and the course begins.

When Pichest is asked who his teachers are, he always mentions the Buddha, Dr. Shivago (Jivaka Kumar Bhaccha), the yogi spirit, and his father. He also often adds Kruba Sri Wichai, Chiangmai's patron saint; Professor Dol Jai, who taught at Wat Po and at the Old Medicine Hospital; and a man named Lung Ta who lived in Hang Dong and taught Pichest to read the old northern Thai language so that he could read a book given to him by Professor Dol Jai.

Pichest stresses that meditation is the most important practice in his life and that it has taught him so much, including ways to improve his teaching and massage practice. He often mentions that he would like to become a monk.

I once asked him what he would wish for if he could have what he most wanted. Without a moment's hesitation he said, "To be able to help as many people as possible." I was very touched. All of us who have studied with Pichest recognize the great love that he has. It is that and his wonderful smile that remain with one even if all of the massage techniques are forgotten.

Now, years later, the little boy who used to walk on his father's back has an international group of students studying under him in the little village of Hang Dong.

*Therefore, a kind heart and compassion are the real
sources of peace and happiness.*

—His Holiness The Dalai Lama

NOTES

Chapter 1 Massage: Compassion in Action

1. Clyde W. Ford, *Where Healing Waters Meet: Touching Mind and Emotion through the Body* (Barrytown, NY: Station Hill Press, 1989), p. 12.

Chapter 2 Massage: East and West

1. Wataru Ohashi, *Do-It-Yourself Shiatsu* (New York: Penguin USA, 2001), p. 10.

Chapter 3 Thai Massage: A Unique Style

1. James Nelson Riley, Fred L. Mitchell, Jr., and Dan Bensky, *Thai Manual Medicine as Represented in the Wat Pho Epigraphies; Preliminary Comparison* (South Salem, NY: Redgrave Publishing Company, 1981), p. 181.
2. Terry Clifford, *Tibetan Buddhist Medicine and Psychiatry: The Diamond Healing* (York Beach, ME: Samuel Weiser, Inc., 1984), p. 68.
3. Ibid., p. 69.
4. Ryokyu Endo, *Tao Shiatsu* (New York: Japan Publications, Inc., 1995), pp. 25–27.
5. *Taber's Cyclopedic Medical Dictionary* (Philadelphia: F.A. Davis Company, 1985), p. 133.
6. Lucy Lidell, with Lucy L. Narayani and Giris Rabinovitch, *The Sivananda Companion to Yoga* (London, England: Simon & Schuster, 1983), p. 10.

CHAPTER 4 THE HISTORICAL ROOTS OF THAI MASSAGE

1. J. E. Spencer, *Asia, East by South: A Cultural Geography* (New York: John Wiley & Sons, 1954), p. 22.
2. David Christian, "Silk Roads or Steppe Roads: The Silk Roads in World History," *Journal of World History* Vol. 11, No. 1 (Spring 2000), p. 2.
3. Terry Clifford, *Tibetan Buddhist Medicine and Psychiatry: The Diamond Healing* (York Beach, ME: Samuel Weiser, Inc., 1984), p. 39.
4. David Frawley, *Yoga and Ayurveda* (Delhi, India: Motilal Banarsidas Publishers, 2000), p. 161.
5. Frank Ros, *The Lost Secrets of Ayurvedic Acupuncture* (Delhi, India: Motilal Banarsidas Publishers, 1995), p. xii.
6. Joe Cummings and Steve Martin, *Thailand* (Footscray, Victoria, Australia: Lonely Planet Publications, 2001), p. 19.

CHAPTER 5 THE PHILOSOPHICAL FOUNDATIONS OF THAI MASSAGE

1. David Frawley, *Yoga and Ayurveda* (Delhi, India: Motilal Banarsidas Publishers, 2000), p. 39.
2. Frank Ros, *The Lost Secrets of Ayurvedic Acupuncture* (Delhi, India: Motilal Banarsidas Publishers, 1995), p. 77.
3. The Dalai Lama, *The Tibetan Medical and Astrological Institute Journal* (Dharamsala, Himachal Pradesh, India: The Tibetan Medical and Astrological Institute, July 1995), p. II.
4. James Nelson Riley, Fred L. Mitchell, Jr., and Dan Bensky, *Thai Manual Medicine as Represented in the Wat Po Epigraphies; Preliminary Comparison* (South Salem, NY: Redgrave Publishing Company, 1981), p. 161.

CHAPTER 8 PREPARATION FOR THE SESSION

1. Susan-Jane Beers, *Jamu* (Hong Kong, China: Periplus Editions [HK] Ltd., 2001), p. 103.
2. The Dalai Lama, *Generating the Mind of Enlightenment* (Dharamsala Himachal Pradesh, India: Cho Yang, 1994), p. 4.
3. Terry Clifford, *Tibetan Buddhist Medicine and Psychiatry: The Diamond Healing* (York Beach, ME: Samuel Weiser, 1984), pp. 78–79.
4. Thomas Hanna, *Somatics* (Cambridge, MA: Perseus Books, 1988), p. 33.

CHAPTER 9 THE TRADITIONAL SEQUENCE

1. Ryokyu Endo, *Tao Shiatsu* (New York: Japan Publications, 1995).
2. Maxine Shapiro, *The Dancing Meditation of Thailand Traditional Massage* (Newton, MA: Acupuncture & Healing Therapies, 2000), p. 90.

GLOSSARY

asana. Sanskrit word meaning "yoga posture."

chakra. A spinning energy center in the body.

channel. According to the Chinese definition, this is a passage in the human body in which blood and chi circulate.

chedi. A Thai relic monument.

chi. Chinese word for "vital energy." Also spelled *qi*.

dharma. For Hindus, one's duty in this lifetime; for Buddhists, the realization and teachings of the Buddha.

hara. Japanese term for the abdominal area, where one's center of gravity and vital energy is.

jing. Chinese word for "channels."

ki. Japanese word for "vital energy."

kundalini. Latent spiritual energy.

luo. Chinese word for collaterals, or branches off of the main trunk.

lom. Thai word for "wind," which signifies energy.

nadi. Indian word for energy pathways in the body. It literally means "streams."

nuad. Thai word meaning "massage."

nuad boran. Thai term meaning "ancient massage."

onkkulee. Thai term for a measurement equal to one finger phalange (segment) of the index finger, approximately one inch.

prana. Indian Sanskrit word for "vital energy."

qi. *See* chi.

sen. Energy line in Thai massage.

sutra. Discourse attributed to the Buddha and his early followers.

tan den. The point in the hara where the center of ki is.

wai khru. Thai prayer in honor of one's teacher.

wat. Buddhist temple in Thailand.

BIBLIOGRAPHY

Brust, Harold. *The Art of Traditional Thai Massage.* Bangkok, Thailand: Editions Duang Kamol, 1990.

Brust, Harold. *Thai Traditional Massage for Advanced Practitioners.* Bangkok, Thailand: Editions Duang Kamol, 1996.

Christian, David. "Silk Roads or Steppe Roads: The Silk Roads in World History." *Journal of World History* Vol. 11, No. 1 (Spring 2000), p. 2.

Clifford, Terry. *Tibetan Buddhist Medicine and Psychiatry: The Diamond Healing.* York Beach, ME: Samuel Weiser, Inc., 1984.

Dalai Lama. *The Path to the Enlightenment.* Delhi, India: Motilal Banarsidas Publishers, 1995.

Dalai Lama. *The Path to Tranquility: Daily Wisdom.* New York: Penguin Books, 1978.

Donden, Yeshi. *Health Through Balance.* Ithaca, NY: Snow Lion Publications, 1986.

Endo, Ryokyu. *Tao Shiatsu.* New York: Japan Publications, 1995.

Ford, Clyde. *Where Healing Waters Meet: Touching Mind and Emotion Through the Body.* Barrytown, NY: Station Hill Press, 1989.

Frawley, David. *Yoga & Ayurveda.* Delhi, India: Motilal Banarsidas Publishers, 2000.

Govindan, S.V. *Massage for Health and Healing.* New Delhi, India: Shakti Malik, 1996.

James, Anthony. *Nuat Thai Traditional Thai Medical Massage the Northern Style.* Chicago: Metta Journal Press, 1993.

Lidell, Lucy, with Narayani and Giris Rabinovitch. *The Sivananda Companion to Yoga.* London, England: Simon & Schuster, 1983.

Lycholat, Tony. *The Complete Book of Stretching.* Ramsbury, Marlborough, England: The Crowood Press, 1990.

Mercati, Maria. *Thai Massage.* London, England: Marshall Publishing, 1998.

Namikoshi, Toru. *Shiatsu and Stretching.* New York: Japan Publications, USA, 1985.

Ohashi, Wataru. *Do-It-Yourself Shiatsu.* New York: Penguin USA, 2001.

Ros, Frank. *The Lost Secrets of Ayurvedic Acupuncture.* Delhi, India: Motilal Banarsidas Publishers, 1995.

Sergel, David. *The Macrobiotic Way of Zen.* New York: Japan Publications, USA, 1989.

Shapiro, Maxine. *The Dancing Meditation of Thailand Traditional Massage.* Newton, MA: Acupuncture & Healing Therapies, 2000.

Shealy, C. Norman. *The Complete Illustrated Encyclopedia of Alternative Healing Therapies.* Boston: Element Books Limited, 1999.

Subcharoen, Pennapa. *The History and Development of Thai Traditional Medicine.* Bangkok, Thailand: National Institute of Thai Traditional Medicine, 1995.

Tapanya, Sombat. *Traditional Thai Massage.* Bangkok, Thailand: Editions Duang Kamal, 1990.

Van Lysebeth, Andre. *Yoga Self-Taught.* New York: Harper & Row, 1968.

Wat Po. *Thai Traditional Massage.* Bangkok, Thailand: Wat Po, 1992.

CREDITS

The photographs on pages iv, 1, 29, and 249 and the drawings on pages 79, 87, 130, 138, and 163 are by Ananda Apfelbaum.

The drawings on pages 12, 40, 43, 44, 46, 47, 48, 88, 94, 151, 157, and 190 are by Tan Waphat.

The maps on pages 20, 21, and 30 are by Henry Kaufman.

The photograph on page 53 is by Heidi Kettler.

The photographs on pages 57–61, 75, 77, 78, 80–83, 85, 89–217, 219, and 223–248 are by Anna Isaak-Ross.

The drawings on pages 136, 137, 171, and 172 are by Joan Berry.

The photographs on pages 126, 210, 218 and 220–222 are by Christian Schubert.

RESOURCES

Mats

Thai Yoga Healing Arts
Jonas Westring
318 Silver Street
Bennington, VT 05201
917-842-9026
info@thaiyogahealing.com
www.thaiyogahealing.com
Thai Bodywork futon mats for Thai massage.

YogaMats
P.O. Box 885044
San Francisco, CA 94188
800-720-YOGA (800-720-9462)
www.yogamats.com
Mats, bolsters, pillows, blocks, and accessories.

Instructional Video

Traditional Thai Massage Center
Ananda Apfelbaum
92 Foster Street
Littleton, MA 01460
978-486-3440

ananda@traditionalthaiyogamassage.com
www.traditionalthaiyogamassage.com
Thai massage video showing a whole-body treatment.

PLACES TO STUDY THAI MASSAGE
UNITED STATES AND CANADA

Acupuncture and Healing Therapies
Maxine Shapiro
53 Marshall Street
Newton, MA 02459-1657
617-965-5251
thai@shortcuts.com
http://health.shortcuts.com

The Center for Thai Yoga Therapy
Saul David Raye
P.O. Box 903
Topanga, CA 90290
310-313-5076
info@thaiyoga.com
www.thaiyoga.com

Institute of Thai Massage—USA
Rose Griscom
P.O. Box 1272
Boynton Beach, FL 33425-1272
561-547-9340
rose@thai-massage.org
http://thai-massage.org

International Professional School of Body Work
Pacific College of Oriental Medicine
Richard Gold
San Diego, CA
800–748-6497
rmgold@znet.com

Lotus Palm School
Kam Thye Chow

1024 Fairmount Ouest
Outremont, QC H2V 267
Canada
514-270-5713
lotuspalm@hotmail.com
www.lotuspalm.com

Omega Institute
150 Lake Drive
Rhinebeck, NY 12572
800-944-1001
www.eomega.org

Thai Yoga Healing Arts
Jonas Westring
318 Silver Street
Bennington, VT 05201
917-842-9026
info@thaiyogahealing.com
www.thaiyogahealing.com

Traditional Thai Masssage Center
Ananda Apfelbaum
92 Foster Street
Littleton, MA 01460
978-486-3440
ananda@traditionalthaiyogamassage.com
www.traditionalthaiyogamassage.com

EUROPE

The School of Thai Yoga Massage
Kira Balaskas
P.O. Box 33822
London N8 8XA
0845-0900-211
info@thaiyogamassage.co.uk
www.thaiyogamassage.co.uk

Thailand

Pichest Boonthumme
3/3 M. 5 T. Bahn Vehn A.
Hang Dong, Chiangmai 50230
Thailand
66-53-441704

Old Medicine Hospital
78/1 Wualai Road (across from Old Chiangmai Cultural Center)
Chiangmai 50100
Thailand
66-53-275085

Asokananda
Sunshine Guest House
149, Kaew Nawarat Soi 4
Chiangmai 50000
Thailand
ashokasunshine@hotmail.com
http://thaiyogamassage.infothai.com

Institute for Thai Massage
17/7 Morakot Road
Hah Yaek Santitham
Chiangmai
Thailand
66-53-218632

Lek Chaiya Nerve-Touch Massage
9/12 Hatsadisaewee Road Sriphum
Chiangmai 50200
Thailand
66-53-404253

Wat Po Thai Traditional Medical School
Sanamachai Road, Wat Po
Bangkok 10200
Thailand
66-2-2254771 or 66-2-2212874

BRIEF BIOGRAPHIES

The following are brief biographical sketches of two individuals who helped in the creation of this book, and to whom I wish to extend special thanks.

Anna Isaak-Ross, Photographer

Anna Isaak-Ross is a graduate of Syracuse University's School of Visual and Performing Arts. She lives in New York City and works as a freelance photographer, designer, and sculptor. Anna is currently working in a style that merges her photography and sculpture using alternative processes. She has exhibited in New York and Massachusetts. She can be contacted at annair@earthlink.net.

Ganitha Manepakorn Notman, Model

Ganitha Notman is from the Isaan region of northeast Thailand. She studied Thai massage with many people, including her grandmother with whom she studied when she was a little girl. More recently, she studied at Wat Pho as well as with other teachers in Chiangmai and with Mae Hong

Son. Most important, however, Ganitha was among the first group of Thai students to take part in an 800-hour program sponsored by the Thai government to revive and pass on the traditional healing arts of Thailand. Ganitha is currently practicing in Portland, Maine, and in Marion, Massachusetts. She can be contacted at dnotman@yahoo.com.

ABOUT THE AUTHOR:
MY STORY

I was born in America. When I was eleven, I went to India with my family for a transformative two years. During my first year there, I went to a public school. One day after school I noticed many of my classmates going to dance class. I asked the teacher if I could join them. He nodded, pleased that a foreign girl was interested in learning classical Indian dance.

When I was twelve, I left the school but continued studying under my dance teacher for another year. He came to our home every week and taught me and my two sisters. In addition to the dance, he introduced us to Indian philosophy and told us stories about all kinds of things such as spirit possession, the Hindu gods and goddesses, and the miraculous cleansing affect of the Ganges river.

When we returned to the United States, I begged my parents to find me another dance teacher. Luckily, they found an Indian woman living in Brookline, Massachusetts, who was a dancer. Every week I took a bus and a train to the city for my dance class. This continued all the way through high school.

At graduation, the big question was what I would do. I had three main interests—prison reform work, photography, and filmmaking. I got an evening-shift job at a pizza place so that I could film in the daytime. Then one night I had a vision and knew that I had to go back to India for spiritual development, which was to come through dance. I worked hard, saving all my money from house painting and restaurant work. Eventually, I flew off to India. I found a good dance teacher and later joined a dance college. The search for a spiritual teacher continued but in a quieter way.

I continued studying dance and later taught and performed until I was 28. At that time I was in the States after a long period in India and I realized that my hearing had declined. I had been born with a neurosensory hearing loss, but the doctors had told my family that it would never get worse. It turned out they were wrong. Overnight, I felt my world turn upside down. Now the doctors were saying that my hearing would progressively degenerate. I quit dancing, worried that my future as a dancer would be too difficult as I needed to hear the music. What could I do if I became deaf? What profession would use my understanding of the body and be compassionate? Massage came to my mind and I enrolled in massage school.

It was the shiatsu training that really spoke to me. I liked the movements and working on the mat. I decided to go to Japan for further training and booked a ticket. A few weeks before my scheduled departure, I was poring over a shiatsu magazine and noticed an article on Thai massage. The photos in the article excited me, as so much movement was shown. I called the author of the article. He was very encouraging and gave me the names of people to study with in Chiangmai, northern Thailand. I decided to change my ticket to Japan for a ticket to Thailand.

I remember my first night in Chiangmai. My hotel window looked out onto an arched temple roof that was glittering in the moonlight. It was sheer magic. Wonderful days followed with Thai massage classes, delicious food, and heartwarming contacts. I was happy to be there. Later, I went to Japan for shiatsu training, which was invaluable, but it was the dancelike movements of Thai massage that called me.

I returned to Thailand, and after studying with many different teachers, I was fortunate to reconnect with a wonderful teacher named Pichest Boonthumme, with whom I have studied ever since. Watching him is like watching beautiful dance choreography. There is such grace and dynamism. Also a very tangible spiritual energy seems to envelop the room when he works.

Later on in my life, I was fortunate to meet and receive teachings from His Holiness The Dalai Lama. In 1997, out of my gratitude and concern for the Tibetan situation, I set up the Tibetan Relief Project, a nonprofit organization to help destitute Tibetans. I am still running this organization today. I am also dancing again, although this time traditional Tibetan dance. Nowadays, I divide my time between Thai massage and my Tibetan involvements. They seem to go hand in hand. I offer this book to each of you who is traveling down the path of compassion and wishes to make this world a more peaceful place.

Only a spontaneous feeling of empathy with others can really inspire us to act on their behalf. Nevertheless, compassion does not arise mechanically. Such a sincere feeling must grow gradually, cultivated within each individual, based on their own conviction of its worth. Adopting a kind attitude thus becomes a personal matter. How each of us behaves in daily life is, after all, the real test of compassion.

—His Holiness The Dalai Lama

ACKNOWLEDGMENTS

My deepest thanks to the many, many, many people who made this book possible: Pichest Boonthumme, who shared his art with me; Bren Jacobsen, for being a great agent; Glen Black, for his generous and expert anatomy help; Bill Williams, for his very inspiring and generous explanations of how the body works; Art Steinhauer for generous legal help; Henry Kaufman, for the beautiful maps; Lori Brungard, for the loan of many books; Aftab Becket, for heartfelt support throughout the process; Anna Isaak-Ross, for great photography and tremendous help pulling the book together; Christian Schubert, for his photography and a very generous heart; Ophiel, for tremendous computer help; Kareema, for rescuing me when I had computer questions; Mary Bloom, for the generous loan of her photographic backdrop; Clemens Kalischer and Jim Higgins, for their kind loan of photo equipment; Omega Institute, for letting me practice and teach there for many years; the Abode of the Message, for supporting my writing retreat in so many ways; Joan Berry, for her drawings and support; Jean Leplante, for her generosity in the bookstore; Pamela Herrick, for helping me long distance while she was in Thailand; Rungrat Pawaradisan, for her friendship and healing when I was in Thailand; my family and Penpa Tsering, for their loving support through the process; Anne Cairns, for her thoughtful listening and good ideas; and the many other people along the way who helped this book come to completion.